The
WEIGHT
of the
NATION

The
WEIGHT
of the
NATION

Surprising Lessons About

DIETS, FOOD, and **FAT**

from the Extraordinary Series from

HBO DOCUMENTARY FILMS®

St. Martin's Press

New York

THE WEIGHT OF THE NATION. Copyright © 2012 by Home Box Office, Inc. and the National Academy of Sciences. All rights reserved. Printed in the United States of America. For information, address St. Martin's Press, 175 Fifth Avenue, New York, N.Y. 10010.

www.stmartins.com

HBO and related service marks are the property of Home Box Office, Inc. *Weight of the Nation* is a trademark owned by the U.S. Department of Health and Human Services (DHHS/CDC), and is used under license. Use of this trademark is not an endorsement by DHHS/CDC of a particular company or organization.

ISBN 978-1-250-01473-3 (hardcover)
ISBN 978-1-250-01474-0 (e-book)

First Edition: April 2012

10 9 8 7 6 5 4 3 2 1

Contents

Contents

Acknowledgments

We would like to begin by thanking Heather Maclean for her significant contributions to this book.

We also would like to recognize the many contributions of our partners, the Centers for Disease Control and Prevention and the National Institutes of Health, with whom we worked on the development and production of the HBO series, *The Weight of the Nation*. We are especially indebted to the Michael & Susan Dell Foundation and Kaiser Permanente for all their collaboration and for their support of a national public health campaign to extend the reach of the HBO series and this book.

We are grateful to the senior management of HBO and the Institute of Medicine of the National Academy of Sciences. In particular, we would like to recognize HBO's Chairman, Bill Nelson; Richard Plepler, Co-President; Sheila Nevins, Documentary Films President; and Michael Lombardo, Programming President, for fostering an environment that allows projects like *The Weight of the Nation* to

Acknowledgments

flourish. At the Institute of Medicine (IOM), we would like to recognize Dr. Harvey V. Fineberg, President; James Hinchman, National Research Council Deputy Executive Officer; and the dedicated program staff of the IOM for their unwavering support of this project. We would also like to thank all those at HBO and the National Academy of Sciences who have gone above and beyond in their efforts to make *The Weight of the Nation* a success.

Additional thanks to everyone who helped shape our thinking about the obesity epidemic and the science of weight loss, as well as to all the people who so generously allowed us to share their stories.

Special thanks to the following people for their contributions to the research, writing, and editing of this book: Nazenet Habtezghi, Tomek Gross, and Sonia Dulay Ricci at HBO; and Linda Meyers, Lynn Parker, and Emily Ann Miller at the IOM. We are also grateful to Bill Dietz and his team at the CDC for lending their expertise.

Finally, we would like to thank the dedicated team at St. Martin's Press: Elizabeth Beier, Michelle Richter, Amelie Littell, Eric C. Meyer, Eliani Torres, Rowen Davis, Jason Ramirez, Matt Baldacci, John Murphy, Laura Clark, and Nadea Mina; and recognize the work of HBO's agent, Brian Lipson.

—John Hoffman and Judith A. Salerno

Foreword

At first glance, body weight seems simple to understand—people eat more than they burn off through physical activity, and their weight goes up. The remedy seems simple as well—push away from the table, exercise, and take some responsibility. There is some truth to each of these propositions, but they both skirt the most important questions:

- Why do so many people struggle with their weight if the problem is so simple?
- What in the world can be done?

If one scratches just below the surface, it quickly becomes apparent that obesity is one of the most fascinating and vexing problems of modern life. A half century ago, obesity was scarce. Then it was a problem only in a few developed countries such as the United States, England, and Australia. Then it stampeded throughout the world. Who would have imagined the day when overnutrition and obesity would join hunger as a leading nutrition problem in countries such as China and India?

Something profound has changed to cause this. A combination of conditions has eroded the ability of vast numbers of people to make healthy choices, even though most people know the rudiments of healthy living—most people know that fruits and vegetables are good and junk food is bad, and that exercise is beneficial. What is driving these problems?

This book answers that question, but it also goes further. It provides sound advice for people wanting to lose weight and keep it off. Based on groundbreaking films produced by HBO in conjunction with the prestigious Institute of Medicine, this book shows that forces working against us make obesity an understandable, even predictable consequence of our environment. The chapter titles capture the daunting challenges people face in everyday life: "Fast Food vs Us," "Restaurants vs Us," "Big Food Companies vs Us," "Marketing vs Us," "Desks, Cars, and Computers vs Us," and so on. The authors show how an environment of toxic food and low physical activity has led us to an epidemic, and they do so in a most accessible and vibrant way.

At the end of the day, the most important challenge is discovering what to do about obesity. Many parties must take part: governments, schools, the media, health professionals, food companies, and, of course, individuals. Individuals can become political actors and cry out to their elected leaders for needed change. Individuals can also address their own behavior and their family environment. This combination of activating people to have a voice and also to adopt new healthy eating and activity patterns is what makes this book unique and so important.

John Hoffman and Judith A. Salerno have made a compelling case for the benefits of weight loss, even in surprisingly small amounts. For people wanting to lose weight, this book brings together the most advanced scientific discoveries into an easily understood and engaging set of guidelines and suggestions designed to bring about sustainable personal change. This information will be helpful to every reader.

It is heartening that *The Weight of the Nation* is also addressing the issue of weight bias, stigma, and discrimination. Overweight people are treated differently from their normal-weight peers in educational, medical, employment, and other settings, even when their qualifications are the same. There is a stunning social penalty for being overweight. And behind the statistics are heart-wrenching stories of children being teased in the cruelest ways by peers, parents being critical of their own children, bullying, and many other forms of mistreatment aimed at people who deserve better.

Some people justify such mistreatment by believing that bias is a form of social pressure that will motivate people to lose weight. Far from the truth, this attitude perpetuates unfair and hurtful behaviors that undermine dignity and good health. It is possible and necessary to fight obesity while showing compassion for the people who have it.

After many years of neglect, governments, public health officials, and society have turned attention to one of the world's most significant public health issues. The result is an amazing series of discoveries, more knowledge than ever about what causes the problem of overweight in America, and more helpful information on how to bring about change. When the history of obesity is written, *The Weight of the Nation* will be seen as a significant milestone.

Kelly D. Brownell, Ph.D.
Professor of Psychology, Epidemiology, and Public Health
Director, Rudd Center for Food Policy & Obesity
Yale University

Introduction

You've heard it a million times: America is fat. As a nation, we're getting fatter every day, our kids are fat, it's making us sick, and many of us may die earlier because of it.

No one is immune. If you're not currently struggling with your weight, you know someone who is, most likely no farther away than your immediate family. The obesity problem in America affects our already strained health-care system, our national productivity and security, and our quality of life.

We spend more than $40 billion every year on diet products and services, trying *not* to be fat—that's not a little concern, that's more than the GDP of half the world's nations. We *really* don't want to be fat.

So why are we? Why is this problem only getting worse? What are the consequences of this seemingly inexorable weight gain? And can anything be done about it?

These are the questions HBO's Emmy Award–winning documentary film division set out to answer in 2009, when they turned their lens to the obesity crisis. Their first step was to partner with the Institute of Medicine (IOM) of the National Academies, which has studied the obesity epidemic for more than ten years, to help them get to the heart of the issue.

New research is released all the time, shifting the blame from one product to another. The first villain was fat itself, so we looked for lower-fat products. That didn't work. Then we tried blaming carbs, then eggs, then red meat, dairy, white flour, sugar, apple juice, soda, high-fructose corn syrup, and partially hydrogenated anything. One by one, we replaced the evil food du jour . . . and watched as our collective waistlines grew. And kept growing! If current trends continue, by 2018, experts predict that 75 percent of the American population will be overweight or obese.

If we couldn't blame carbs or fat, what was left to blame but ourselves? You ate too much at the holidays: better join a weight-loss program. If you really wanted it bad enough, you'd lose those last ten pounds. You'd actually use that gym membership that hits your credit card bill every month. Unlike our hardworking grandparents, people today are less active, and we indulge at every meal. Could it really be that hard to just eat less and exercise more?

Far too many people look at weight problems and think it should be easy enough to eat less and move more. But if more than two-thirds of American adults are overweight or obese, it can't be so simple. And the notion that we're not strong or smart enough to stop overeating isn't helping anyone. That kind of stigma only makes it more difficult for those of us who are struggling with our weight. It does, however, benefit the diet industry when it needs to sell its latest program, product, or book. In a world that places such a high value on being thin, and where thinness has come to connote a superior level of self-control, those who fail to achieve such an ideal take much of the blame. Popular culture and the media tell us it's as easy as just saying no to unhealthy foods and large portions, and that not being able to do so is a mark of personal failure. That kind of blame game doesn't set anyone up for success. Actually, it undermines many of our best efforts.

The notion that obesity is the result of a lack of willpower or self-control resonated with the HBO documentary film team. In *The Addiction Project*, they'd stared down the same prejudice against those struggling with addiction and successfully reframed it as a chronic, relapsing brain disease for which we have increasingly effective treatments. They cut through the misinformation and fear surrounding dementia and brought hope to a previously desperate diagnosis with *The Alzheimer's Project*. Now, with their immersion into the world of obesity in *The Weight of the Nation*, they've come to understand the powerful mechanisms in our bodies and brains that cause us to gain weight and interfere with losing it. The forces within us that work in ways outside our awareness and beyond our control are so strong that they dwarf any argument that it is all about willpower. There has to be more going on with the obesity story.

HBO was aware that the IOM had already developed an extensive body of work on the prevention of childhood obesity and had a strong desire to raise awareness about this personal and public health problem. IOM's obesity prevention reports consistently emphasized viewing obesity as an enormously complex problem that is much more than an issue of "personal responsibility," and stressed that the environment in which children and families live often makes it very difficult to attain or maintain a healthy weight. The recommendations in its reports focused on the importance of change at every level and the need to motivate and empower individuals and communities to act to turn the tide of the obesity epidemic. The combination of the IOM's in-depth background in obesity prevention research and its focus on solutions made it an excellent partner in helping to tell the obesity story.

Together, HBO and the IOM worked with the National Institutes of Health (NIH), the Centers for Disease Control and Prevention (CDC), the Michael & Susan Dell Foundation, and Kaiser Permanente to gather the nation's leading experts in every field from heart disease and diabetes to evolutionary biology, agriculture, food marketing, and behavioral economics. For more than two years, we examined and analyzed historical and groundbreaking studies. To put a human face on the problem, we interviewed hundreds of people who have struggled with their weight and chronicled their challenges.

The Weight of the Nation is more than a documentary series. It is an ambitious public health campaign consisting of four documentary films, a series of films for children, a video-rich Web site at hbo.com/theweightofthenation, the free distribution of forty thousand screening kits to organizations around the country, and action-oriented community-based outreach efforts. Together, all this adds up to a comprehensive campaign to reverse obesity in America—the latest word on the consequences of being fat, why we gain weight, how to lose it, and the best ways of keeping weight off.

PART I

||||||||||||||||||||||||||||||||||

Good News and Bad News

1

The Bad News:
We Have a Big Problem

As much as we all wish there were one thing in the fight against fat we could point to and eliminate, there isn't. Whether you look at individuals or at our society as a whole, the cause is complex. It's the sum total of all our little daily decisions that results in us eating a little too much and moving too little—which over time adds up to a lot of pounds. For the nation, our obesity problem has been magnified by the actions of industry, agriculture, and government. These forces shape the environment in which we live, work, and play and, often unintentionally, make it harder for us to make healthy choices. Big decisions made by industry, agriculture, and government have a huge impact on the little decisions we make about what we reach for when we're hungry and how long we sit at our desks and in our cars.

The good news is that, to some extent, there are things within our control that we can change to help ourselves, our families, and our communities pursue healthier lives.

Obesity is not inevitable. It *can* be prevented. And, with hard work and the right information, it can even be reversed.

We Know We're Fat . . . Don't We?

Our national obsession with stick-thin beauty as portrayed in television shows, movies, and magazines has confused an entire generation about what healthy actually looks like. But, equally concerning are the generations of Americans who now look at the overweight and obese people around them and mistake them for people who are at a normal size and a healthy weight.

So, if our perspective is so distorted, how can we tell when our fat is an actual problem and not just a bothersome muffin top?

How Fat Is Too Fat?

If you're cutting through the fat to try to figure that question out, what are the most important measurements you need to pay attention to? The simple answer is your waist size and your body mass index. The bigger your waist, the more likely you are to be storing an unhealthy amount of fat in your abdomen. Excess fat that accumulates in your midsection is directly associated with your risk of developing the chronic health conditions linked to obesity, so waist size is a critical measurement to know. A quick and fairly accurate way to measure it is as simple as stretching a piece of string around your stomach. Find the circumference of your bare waist just above your hipbones. Men who measure at over forty inches and (non-pregnant) women who measure over thirty-five inches are at risk.

One of the terms that gets used most often in discussions about obesity, weight loss, and weight gain is body mass index, or BMI, which is a ratio of weight and height that represents how much body fat you have. The most important thing you need to know about BMI is that it's the calculation most often used by your physician. It's also valuable to scientists and statisticians, because it's a reliable measure that is easy to figure out. Because BMI is so commonly used, it's crucial to know what yours is. The standard BMI chart is broken down into the following categories:

ADULT (20 years+) BMI CHART	
Underweight	Less than 18.5
Healthy Weight	18.5–24.9
Overweight	25.0–29.9
Obese	30 and above
Morbidly Obese	40 and above
Calculate your own BMI at hbo.com/theweightofthenation.	

WHAT IS FAT?

Adipose tissue, the scientific name for body fat, is required for human development and survival. We all need fat for energy storage, metabolism, growth, brain function, temperature insulation, organ protection, and structural cushioning. (Imagine sitting without it!) But adipose tissue is not the only place fat cells live. They're everywhere in your body—in your organs and even in your blood.

The number of fat cells each person has varies: a lean person has around 40 billion, an obese adult might have 120 billion. How many you end up with depends on many things, including genetics, but scientists believe there are three times in your life when you can make a lot of them—the third trimester just before you're born, the first year of life, and during puberty.

Once you've made fat cells and settled at a number, here's the bad news: That number can never get lower again. When you lose weight, you're actually not losing any fat cells. The ones you have are just shrinking. An obese person not only has up to three times more fat cells than someone at a healthy weight who's never been obese, but their fat cells themselves can be twice as large as the fat cells of a lean person. Lose weight, though, and the cells will contract.

When you consume excess calories and the body has no more empty fat cells to fill, the only thing it can do to store them is to make more fat cells. Many of the health problems that result from the production of these additional fat cells are caused by the fact that they are not just under your skin. They are also accumulating inside your abdomen, where they surround your internal organs, and, amazingly and dangerously, within some of those organs, like the liver and the heart. When fat begins to accumulate inside your organs, it dangerously disrupts your metabolism.

To be healthy, the body of an average (read: non-marathoner) adult woman should be about 21 to 31 percent fat. The body of a healthy, average (read: non–NFL linebacker) adult male should be roughly between 14 and 24 percent fat.

Still, BMI isn't a perfect measurement of our body fat or of our risk for related health conditions. For example, highly competitive athletes tend to have higher BMIs because of increased muscle mass. For the vast majority of us, though, our BMI reflects our level of body fat and our health risks. While the BMI chart is the same for men and women, BMI calculations for children take into account their growth and development and should be determined by a pediatrician at every visit. If the result concerns you and your doctor, you should discuss both its implications and what you can do to help your child.

What may surprise you is that you don't need to have a BMI in the obese range to start developing the adverse health outcomes related to carrying too much weight. Being even a few pounds overweight can start you down the path to type 2 diabetes—and you can tip over into type 2 diabetes without ever becoming obese.

The Growing Majority

So how does the rest of the population look?

According to the CDC's most recent survey of America's health, released in January 2012, almost 32 percent of 2- to 19-year-olds and nearly 69 percent of adults in America are overweight or obese.

In 2010, the obesity rate for adults rose in sixteen states. And how many states saw a decrease? None. While it's true the rate of increase has begun to slow, that doesn't mean we're out of the woods yet.

The obesity epidemic is like a flood. The rush of water may have abated, but our nation is still more than two-thirds underwater. And in some demographic groups and income brackets, the floodwaters are still pouring in. Ever since 2005, there is no longer a linear relationship between poverty and obesity. Being wealthy is not nearly as protective against obesity as it used to be.

Being overweight or obese isn't just uncomfortable—it's also deadly, as obesity is far too often followed by a wave of chronic disease. But the obesity epidemic is not a natural disaster that we can't do anything about. Unlike a tsunami, this national crisis is completely preventable.

2

The Worse News:
It's Making Us Sick

Collectively, Americans carry more than four and a half billion extra pounds—that's an average of fourteen and a half pounds per person. This excess body fat, whether it accumulates under our skin, around our abdomens, or inside our organs, wreaks havoc on our bodies, which are simply not designed to carry all that extra weight. As a result, obesity is a culprit behind the countless chronic diseases affecting us today. According to CDC estimates, obesity is associated with approximately 112,000 deaths each year.

Heart Broken

Did you know that every twenty-five seconds someone in this country has a heart attack? This alarming statistic accounts for heart disease's rank as the number one cause of death for both men and women. More people die from heart-related problems than from cancer, AIDS, respiratory disease, or even accidents. And if you are obese or overweight, you are more likely to have high blood pressure, high levels of triglycerides and LDL ("bad") cholesterol, and low levels of HDL ("good") cholesterol, all of which are risk factors for heart disease. The bottom line: Being overweight or obese places you at a higher risk of developing heart disease and stroke.

According to Dr. Donald Lloyd-Jones, the chair of preventive medicine at Northwestern University, we shouldn't be surprised by this. "The heart is a muscle like any other in our body," he explains. But there's one important exception: "It never gets to rest." Your heart—the hardest-working muscle—spends every second of every day vigorously pumping blood to the farthest reaches of your body. The larger you become, the harder your heart has to work to keep blood circulating. The heart's smooth muscle walls start to thicken and get bigger. According to Dr. Lloyd-Jones, "pretty quickly the thickened heart starts to weaken and eventually tips over into heart failure."

Clogged Pipes

Arteries are the smooth, elastic vessels that transport blood throughout the body. When you have high levels of LDL, the "bad" cholesterol, it can stick to inflamed sections of the artery walls and eventually build up into deposits called plaques. Just as gunk in the drain of your sink would prevent water from flowing out of the basin and down the pipe, causing a backup, clogged arteries reduce blood flow, increasing the risk of a heart attack or stroke. If a coronary artery is completely blocked off, it interrupts the blood supply to the heart muscle, causing what we know as a heart attack.

For many of us, there is a genetic component to cholesterol beyond our control that cannot be overlooked. If your cholesterol is too high despite being at a healthy weight and eating a healthy diet, there are other ways to reduce it. The discovery and wide use of statin drugs (like Lipitor and its generics) have been a boon to the heart health of our nation. With changes in diet and drug-induced reductions of further buildup of plaque in the arteries, you can dramatically reduce your risk of heart attack and stroke.

A High-Pressure Situation

As the heart pumps harder with increased body size and the arteries narrow with elevated cholesterol, blood pressure almost inevitably begins to climb. High blood pressure, also known as hypertension, is a major risk factor for heart disease and stroke. Sixty-nine percent of people suffering their first heart attack and 74 percent of stroke victims have high blood pressure. The most common contributors to high blood pressure line up perfectly with the modern American lifestyle: being overweight, not engaging in enough physical activity, and eating a poor diet high in sodium.

UNDER PRESSURE

High blood pressure is not only a leading cause of heart disease and stroke in this country, but a leading cause of kidney disease as well. Sustained high blood pressure damages blood vessels throughout the body, and the small vessels that provide blood to our kidneys are especially vulnerable. If those vessels are compromised, the kidneys may stop removing waste and extra fluid from the body. That extra fluid can then raise blood pressure even further, and the health problems only mount.

If enough damage accumulates in the kidneys, it can lead to kidney failure (also called end-stage renal disease). The only treatments for kidney failure are dialysis, which means having to undergo regular blood-cleaning treatments for the rest of your life, and kidney transplant, which is a procedure with its own drawbacks and risks. High blood pressure causes more than twenty-five thousand new cases of kidney failure in this country every year.

7 Steps to a Healthy Heart

Wonder what makes for ideal cardiovascular health and whether you meet the criteria? Give your heart a break and show it some love by trying to check off as many of these American Heart Association factors as possible:

1. Optimal cholesterol (less than 200 mg/dL)
2. Normal blood pressure (120/80 or lower)
3. Not having diabetes
4. Lean body mass index (BMI of less than 25)
5. Not smoking
6. Physical activity
7. Healthy diet

Unfortunately, according to the American Heart Association, only 1 percent of American adults meet these criteria. To find out how many you meet, go to mylifecheck.heart.org.

The United States of Diabetes

TYPE 1 VS TYPE 2

Type 1 Diabetes

Was previously known as juvenile diabetes because it is the type that developed most often in childhood. It is not related to obesity, and occurs when the body's immune system destroys the insulin-producing cells so insulin therapy is required.

Type 2 Diabetes

Develops when the body can't use insulin properly or no longer makes enough of it to overcome insulin resistance. It most often affects overweight and older adults, and accounts for approximately 90 percent of people with diabetes.

High blood sugar, the telltale sign of diabetes, is caused by the body's failure to move glucose out of the bloodstream and into the cells, where it is used for energy. Carrying too much weight, especially when fat is concentrated in the abdomen, makes you resistant to your own insulin, the hormone that moves glucose from your blood into your cells. In response, the pancreas works hard to produce ever-higher levels of insulin in an attempt to keep blood glucose levels from rising. Type 2 diabetes ultimately ensues when the body's cells become resistant to insulin and thus cannot properly remove glucose from the bloodstream. And, in some cases, the insulin-producing cells of the pancreas eventually become exhausted, requiring people with type 2 diabetes to take injections of insulin.

Type 2 diabetes affects nearly 27 million Americans and is inextricably linked with obesity: 80 percent of people with type 2 diabetes are overweight or obese. Currently the seventh-leading cause of death, diabetes, if left untreated or poorly controlled, can contribute to a number of serious health problems, including kidney failure, blindness, and amputations. Unfortunately, the somber stats don't stop there. People with diabetes are up to four times more likely to have a heart attack or stroke than those without it, and 25 percent more likely to die of cancer. The main risk factor for developing type 2 diabetes is weight gain—even going from a BMI of 26 to 27 or 28 can increase your risk substantially.

Type 2 diabetes doesn't develop overnight. More than 79 million Americans are living with a condition called insulin resistance—also known as prediabetes. As we gain weight, our cells become more resistant to insulin, which results in an inability to transport glucose out of the bloodstream as well as we should. This leads to a high blood sugar level, which can be detected by your doctor with a standard panel of blood work. People with prediabetes are at incredibly high risk of tipping over into diabetes in the near future. But since prediabetes has no symptoms, most of the millions of people with prediabetes don't even know they have it, which is one reason it's crucial to have periodic screenings. There are many things that can be done to reverse prediabetes—or even reverse type 2 diabetes—but you can take action only if you know you have a problem. It's believed that more than 90 percent of adults with prediabetes and 25 percent of adults with diabetes don't know they have the disease, because they haven't been tested for it. For more on the different steps you can take, see chapter 3.

Fatty Liver

When you gain too much weight for the body to store it under your skin, it begins to deposit in your belly and eventually spreads out into some of your organs, especially your heart and other muscles—and, most importantly, your liver. Fat deposits in the liver are associated with the metabolic abnormalities that drive the development of both high cholesterol and type 2 diabetes. The growing obesity epidemic has been closely followed by another rising epidemic of this new condition, called nonalcoholic fatty liver disease. Nonalcoholic fatty liver disease didn't even exist until recently. And now it's estimated that as many as 25 percent of American adults have excess fat in their liver.

In some cases, nonalcoholic fatty liver disease progresses into a form of cirrhosis that occurs almost exclusively in people with severe obesity. Almost all liver transplants in this country are performed as a result of cirrhosis, but it used to be that most of that liver failure could be attributed to the effects of alcoholism or hepatitis B and C. Now, however, the number of liver transplants resulting from cirrhosis caused by nonalcoholic fatty liver disease is quickly rising.

The C Word

Obesity doesn't just affect your heart, vascular system, pancreas, and liver; it also increases your risk of developing some types of cancer, including cancers of the colon, kidneys, and esophagus. In women, it is also linked to uterine cancer and postmenopausal breast cancer. Twenty percent of cancer deaths in women and 14 percent in men are related to being overweight or obese.

Brain Drain

One recent study suggests that being overweight or obese in middle age might increase your likelihood of developing dementia later in life, perhaps by as much as 70 percent. According to Dr. Nora Volkow, a neuroscientist and the director of the National Institute on Drug Abuse, obesity "negatively affects the functioning of the human brain."

When researchers have compared the brain activity of obese people with the brain activity of those at a healthy weight, studies have shown decreased activity in the areas of the brain that control cognition.

Other Aches and Pains

More than 66 percent of people with arthritis are overweight or obese. The hypertension with which so many obese people struggle makes them 83 percent more likely to develop kidney disease. Obesity also increases adults' relative risk of health problems such as gallbladder disease, asthma, sleep apnea, and gout.

We know that obesity is a gateway to serious health conditions, but what are the ramifications of having those conditions earlier in life, when your body's still developing?

Won't Somebody Please Think of the Children?

In 1970, less than 5 percent of American children were obese. By 2008, that figure had skyrocketed to more than 17 percent. Add in the kids who are overweight, and the number soars to almost 33 percent. In African American and Hispanic communities it's even higher: 40 percent.

How's the health of those kids? Not so great. The CDC reports that 20 percent of all American teens, and 40 percent of obese teens, have unhealthy cholesterol levels. Autopsy studies have found that 38 percent of obese children and 13 percent of all children show signs of nonalcoholic fatty liver disease. Pediatricians are now being encouraged to pay close attention to the warning signs of hypertension.

And when it comes to diabetes, children typically aren't screened at all. Prior to the rise of obesity in this country, it simply wasn't necessary. Any diabetes seen in children was usually type 1 diabetes (not related to obesity). Type 2 diabetes historically was seen only in adults, and was called adult-onset diabetes. Now that physicians are seeing it in obese children, they had to stop calling it *adult-onset*, but the health risks are the same.

What will happen when these children who are starting their lives with a progressive disease end up on dialysis before the age of thirty? Type 2 diabetes typically cuts the life expectancy of a fifty-year-old by six years. The CDC estimates that a ten-year-old with type 2 diabetes will lose nineteen years of his or her life.

THE BOGALUSA HEART STUDY

For almost forty years, starting in 1973, researchers gathered the vital statistics of a cohort of grade-school children from Bogalusa, Louisiana, following more than sixteen thousand subjects by the time the study was complete. This landmark study was the first to prove that childhood health, including weight, is a good predictor of heart disease in adulthood, and that overweight and obesity begins damaging the cardiovascular system in preschool, much earlier than anyone thought.

A Life Unexpected

There is much speculation—and worry—that the compounding obesity and diabetes crises will actually shorten our national life expectancy. And if that happens, it will be the first time since the rise of modern civilization it occurs not because of natural disaster, famine, or plague, but as the result of chronic diseases.

Whether or not the average life span decreases, the quality of life for many Americans already has. Obesity can deprive those affected by it not only of health, but also of mobility, self-esteem, opportunities, and, in many cases, success and happiness.

THE HIGH COST OF ILLNESS

Obesity isn't just expensive in terms of individual health-care bills. It has a high cost for our entire nation.

We're Less Productive

Eric Finkelstein and other economists at Duke University found that obesity costs America more than $73 billion a year in lost productivity. According to Finkelstein, some companies are moving jobs overseas in large part because they can't afford to insure employees who have extra health risks associated with obesity and its related diseases.

We're Less Secure

Obesity is also a threat to our national security. Every year, approximately 1,200 enlisted members have to leave the military because of their weight, and we're having trouble finding healthy replacements. Between 1995 and 2008, the military was forced to reject more than 140,000 recruits because they were overweight. Today, it's estimated that one in four young Americans do not meet the weight requirement to join the armed forces. If the pool of overweight candidates keeps growing, it could negatively affect our police and fire departments as well.

We Share Higher Health-Care Costs

Obesity costs our nation $150 billion in direct health costs a year and $139 billion in indirect costs. Half of that is paid through Medicare and Medicaid. If we solved our collective weight problem, that money could be spent on schools, police, libraries, or better roads....

Obesity is a national problem, and one that needs national attention in order to fix it. Every person in this country, even those who are currently at a healthy weight, is or will be touched by obesity in some way. It's everyone's problem, and everyone needs to be part of the solution.

3

The Good News: Little Changes Can Make a Big Difference

The bad news and big numbers connected to our national weight crisis tell us that the obesity epidemic cannot be denied or ignored. To reverse the epidemic, it's going to take changes to every sector of society. However, for any of us who are overweight or obese, it was many little decisions adding up over time that got us to the number on the scale this morning. And making many little changes to our lives can help bring our weight down.

Huge Benefits

An important piece of good news is that most of us don't have to lose fifty pounds to start seeing real improvements to our health. Numerous studies have demonstrated that losing just 10 percent of total body weight—for a 200-pound person, that's twenty pounds; for someone who weighs 150 pounds, it's fifteen—is enough to improve a person's overall health. And for some of us, a 10 percent weight loss could be enough to return our BMI to the healthy zone.

Researchers have found that most health benefits of moderate weight loss actually kick in sooner. Losing as little as 5 to 7 percent of your total weight—seven to fourteen pounds in the above examples—lowers blood pressure, improves blood sugar levels, and reduces the risk of type 2 diabetes by 60 percent. Aching joints? Every ten pounds lost removes an average of forty pounds of pressure on your hips, knees, and ankles; alleviates arthritic pain; and can significantly cut the risk of developing osteoarthritis.

Creeping Up and Cutting Back

For most people, weight gain creeps up on them. It doesn't take a three-week all-inclusive cruise or an entire season of tailgate parties to find your jeans no longer button. Just an extra 100 calories a day can pack on considerable pounds over the course of a year. Five years of snacks you don't even remember eating could explain the thirty pounds that just sneaked up on you.

But that little bit, just 100 calories, makes a difference in the long run. How much is 100 calories? In many cases, it's barely a bite: a third of an average bagel, four Hershey's kisses, or a quarter of a Starbucks blueberry streusel muffin.

Dr. Rudy Leibel, a molecular geneticist at Columbia University, says that, like baseball, obesity is a game of inches. After studying the science of weight for thirty years, Leibel believes individuals become obese due to "very small differences in the balance of energy intake and expenditure, extrapolated over long periods of time, years and years."

Happily, the opposite is also true. Cutting just 100 calories a day is a good first step toward gradual weight loss. Eliminating that one afternoon soda, sweet tea, or vitamin water could start you on the journey toward a healthier, thinner you.

Got Sweat?

Contributing to our collective weight gain is the fact that Americans aren't moving like we used to. In 1950, half of Americans had a job that involved physical labor. Today, less than 20 percent of us do, and we don't compensate for that when we're off the clock. Almost 59 percent of adults don't break a sweat in their leisure time. Only 3 percent of adults meet the minimum recommendation for physical activity.

Do you know you need to step up your physical activity, but don't have the time for a Zumba class, the money for a personal trainer, or the stamina to run a 5K? No worries. You don't need to. The recommended amount is less than you might think.

To glean the most important health benefits of physical activity, the average adult needs to engage in thirty minutes of moderate activity, five times a week, and it doesn't have to be thirty minutes all at once: Shorter bouts of ten to fifteen minutes count too. What counts? Take a brisk walk, ride your bike to work, or climb the five flights of stairs up to your office.

Want to go farther, faster? Just fifteen minutes of vigorous aerobic activity—jogging, riding your bike on hills, or playing basketball—five days a week can have similar health benefits.

New research shows that doing resistance training just two days a week not only strengthens bones and muscles, but also boosts your body's good cholesterol, improves cognitive function, lowers the risk of type 2 diabetes, and reduces depression. Weight lifting and yoga both count. How long? Just move your muscles until they're tired—fifteen minutes can do it.

Little Changes = **Big Results**

Cut just 100 calories a day from your normal diet. You don't even have to give something up: just swap it. Switching your morning bagel—even the whole-grain, covered-in-sunflower-seeds kind—to oatmeal can easily eliminate your 100 calories without depriving you of a single bite. If you're the kind of person who thinks it's not breakfast without a bowl of cold cereal, try swapping your granola for Special K and whole milk or 2 percent for skim or 1 percent.

SUCCESS STORIES

When Paul, a video store owner from Boston, was diagnosed with diabetes fifteen years ago, his identical twin, Tim, was prepared for the same fate. After all, they shared the same DNA, and both brothers were overweight: Paul was 220 pounds; Tim weighed in at 200. The only other difference was that Paul had stopped exercising. Tim still played hoops with his friends on Tuesday nights.

Tim signed up for the Diabetes Prevention Program, an NIH-funded study of more than three thousand volunteers who were overweight and had prediabetes. The goal of the study was to determine if a small amount of weight loss—just 7 percent of one's body weight—and an increase in physical activity were enough to prevent high-risk people from developing diabetes.

And what did the study show? Those participants who made lifestyle changes were twice as successful at preventing diabetes than those who just took medicine to prevent it. In fact, over the course of six months in the study, which offered medical supervision and support, Tim lost fourteen pounds and reversed his own prediabetic condition; his blood sugar levels returned to normal. How did he lose the weight? By making small lifestyle changes. He added a little more exercise to his week—he now carries his own clubs when he plays golf—and cut the size of his portions. He still eats meat and his beloved potato chips, but in moderation.

As Dr. David Nathan, the Harvard endocrinologist who led the Diabetes Prevention Program, sums it up, "You don't have to get back to what you weighed in high school. You only need to lose ten or fifteen pounds to improve your chances of preventing diabetes."

The BEST News Ever!

Before we go one page further, hear this clearly: You don't have to achieve rock-hard abs to be healthy. You don't have to be a woman who wears a size 4 or a man who fits into size 30 jeans. You don't have to completely abandon all the foods you love, become a vegan, or work out for six hours a day. You don't have to be perfect. You just have to be healthy. And healthy comes in all shapes and sizes, with curves and dimples and angles and other beautiful identifiers that make us each unique.

Unlike some serious health conditions, obesity can be reversed. Conquer it and you vastly improve your odds of a longer, healthier, happier life.

Although it's hard, it's less complicated than you think. All too often, people give up because they believe it's all or nothing: They think they have to start training for an Ironman competition and eliminate unhealthy food entirely, subsisting on a meager diet of canned tuna, carrots, celery, and the like. You can try that for a while, but it's unhealthy, unrealistic, and virtually impossible for most of us to maintain—especially when our bodies are programmed to be sedentary when we can and to seek out sweets and fats.

The prescription is simple: Eat a bit less and move a bit more. You don't have to have a system or a supplement, a complicated workout regimen or fancy nutritional calculators. You don't need to join a gym or a boot camp or find a personal trainer. The only thing you need is the truth. The truth about why we're fat, and how we can fix it.

And here's the really good news: You've already got it in your hands. Welcome to the anti-diet book.

PART II

||||||||||||||||||||||||||||||||

Why We Are Fat

Americans are more health-conscious than ever before. Since the 1970s, the mortality rate from both cardiovascular disease and stroke has dropped. Stores have more healthy food options; fewer Americans are smoking; and many people regularly monitor their blood pressure and cholesterol levels.

So why are we fat, and getting fatter?

4

Evolutionary History

There's no denying that, as a society, we eat more today than we ate in the past. In the last fifty years, our plates have literally become 30 percent larger, and the portions on them have been supersized. In the 1960s, the average dinner plate was nine inches in diameter. In the 1970s, restaurants upped their dinner plates to ten inches. Today, our at-home dinner plates are twelve inches wide, while some restaurants now serve individual entrées on platters.

Even if our plates and our portions are bigger, we still have free will, right? No one steers your car into the fast-food drive-through lane or forces your daily doughnut down your throat. . . . The whole nation has gotten lazy and lost its willpower. Why else wouldn't we be able to just say no?

Could it be that we're biologically wired to say yes?

A World of Want

Over the course of human evolution, there has never been any reason to limit our food intake. In fact, it's the opposite. Because we need food to survive, we are genetically programmed to love it. According to Dr. Rudy Leibel, the Columbia University molecular geneticist, there may be as many as one hundred genes that favor food-seeking behavior.

Scientists' best estimate is that today's humans are genetically identical to our ancestors who roamed the savanna 150,000 years ago, when the genus *Homo* arose.

The world of our hunter-gatherer ancestors was one of feast and famine: The food supply was dictated by the seasons and susceptible to droughts, flooding, fire, and plagues. Under such conditions, the ability to ingest and store as many calories as possible when food was readily available was of value for survival, especially in anticipation of the oncoming winter.

According to evolutionary biologists, we evolved a system to favor fat deposition as a buffer against times of scarcity. When we encountered a source of food, such as a ripe fruit tree or fresh prey, we replenished our fat stores by consuming as much as we could. According to Dr. Deborah Clegg, a metabolism researcher at the University of Texas–Southwestern, our bodies and brains developed the ability to suppress the feeling of fullness when consuming animal fats. It was rare to bag an antelope, and, without a fridge to store it, we had to eat while we could. Stuffing ourselves silly had a long-term gain: *Survival!*

SKINNY GENES?

Like many people, you may wonder what role genetics plays in all of this. If our parents are heavy, are we doomed to be obese?

And is that because of the genes we inherit or the culture and behaviors we share?

Dr. David Altshuler, a geneticist and endocrinologist at Massachusetts General Hospital, explains: "When it comes to obesity, for the vast majority of people, there's no one gene that makes a difference. There are many, many genes, dozens, perhaps hundreds, each of which has a small effect on obesity in the population, but which add up to a susceptibility, when exposed to this environment we live in, for getting more overweight or not."

Because it was so beneficial to our hunter-gatherer ancestors to eat as much food as they could find and to store excess calories as fat, it shouldn't be surprising that most of us have that behavior and biology encoded in our genes to some extent. But any individual's weight is the result of the interaction of their genetic makeup with the environment they happen to be living in. Dr. Jack Shonkoff, director of Harvard's Center on the Developing Child, explains: "Both nature, by which we mean genes, and nurture, meaning experience, affect each other. And they're inextricably intertwined. Is there a genetic predisposition to obesity? Absolutely. Is obesity caused by an environment and behavior? Absolutely."

The important thing to keep in mind is that, just because it's written in most of our genes, we're not fated to a lifetime of fat. As Dr. Altshuler puts it, "It's not always the person with the best cards who wins the game. What matters is how well you play the hand you're dealt."

So the evolutionary drive has been to seek food constantly, to gorge when it is readily available, and to store those extra calories as fat in order to survive periods of famine. As noted by Clegg, the elegantly designed systems we evolved to favor fat deposition are just as powerful today as they were 150,000 years ago. But in a world full of burger joints, pizza parlors, and vending machines, our biological imperative to store fat whenever we can may instead pose a threat to our survival.

FAT PETS AND ZOO ANIMALS

Amazingly, the obesity epidemic isn't limited to humans. Our pets and zoo animals increasingly have to battle weight gain as well. While animals in the wild put on fat stores to help tide them over through times of scarcity just like our hunter-gatherer ancestors, an obese wild animal is virtually unknown, with the exception of those that live in proximity to humans and eat our discarded food. According to Sir Peter Gluckman, an expert in evolutionary medicine at New Zealand's University of Auckland, "Animals sitting in zoos, as opposed to their native, wild environments, are more likely to become obese and develop the associated complications. Paradoxically, they live much longer, but they also have the same battle with chronic diseases that humans have."

Just like modern humans, animals in captivity live longer than animals in the wild because they are protected from the conflicts, infectious diseases, accidents, and food shortages that characterize life in the wilderness. But they aren't necessarily any healthier. Male chimps in the wild rarely live past thirty, but captive chimps are living long enough to join the AARP—and in addition to developing many of the same ailments that we do as we get older, they are also experiencing rising rates of overweight and obesity.

And the problem is even worse for Fido and Kitty. More than half of American cats and dogs are now overweight or obese, according to a 2011 survey by the Association for Pet Obesity Prevention, and one-fifth of them are 30 percent or more overweight, which qualifies as obese. What can you do if your canine or feline best friend has put on a few too many pounds around the middle? The two most important steps are the same ones you should be taking in your own life: Feed them a healthy diet, paying attention to portion size, and make sure they get enough physical activity. Remember, walking the dog has benefits for both you and your four-legged friend.

For both animals and humans, a sedentary lifestyle in a dog bed, monkey house, or cubicle and ready access to dog chow, bananas, or junk food are a recipe for caloric imbalance and weight gain.

The Evolution of the Omnivore

Evolutionary biologists tell us that before the origin of the genus *Homo,* the diet of our ancestors was most likely vegetarian. Eating a diet rich in fruits and leaves requires a substantial digestive system to process the food into everything the body needs to function. Think of a cow and the four stomachs it needs to transform the grass that is its only natural food source into the impressive beast that it is.

With the emergence of early man, we became omnivores and began to consume more meat. This, along with the discovery of fire and cooking, which Harvard anthropologist Richard Wrangham argues enabled us to extract more nutrients from every morsel, led to the simultaneous development of larger, more energy-demanding brains. With our increasing intelligence, Wrangham theorizes, we became better hunters and gatherers, upping the proportion of meat in our diet and decreasing our reliance on plant matter. Over the millennia, the one hundred or so genes that Rudy Leibel believes govern our drive to eat led us to seek foods that packed the biggest wallop—those high in fat and sugar—because they easily provide fuel to support our needy brains.

Evolutionary biologists theorize that nature demands a trade-off between the length of our guts and the size of our brains. Modern humans have the largest brains relative to our body mass, and think about what has become of our digestive tract: The last remnant of our leaf-and-shoot-crushing gut shriveled up to become our modern appendix. The end result is a highly intelligent species with a metabolism dependent on an omnivorous diet to obtain the required amounts of protein, carbohydrate, fat, and micronutrients.

The Invention of Agriculture

It was only twelve thousand years ago, a blip of time in evolutionary terms, that, after hundreds of thousands of years of nomadic reliance on the whims of nature, humans invented agriculture. Farming allowed us to obtain more energy from plants, seeds, nuts, and fruit and store surplus food for the winter and for times of famine. We also domesticated livestock, increasing the ready availability of meat and introducing dairy products into the human diet for the first time. Still, obesity was rare in agrarian societies, even up until the early twentieth century, presumably because the supply of food was still cyclical and unpredictable and farming demanded tremendous physical effort.

Agriculture tied people to the land they cleared, planted, and harvested, freeing a portion of this newborn civilization from the daily labors associated with obtaining food and allowing for the growth of cities. It marks the first time in human history that we were able to radically transform our environment, and it set in motion the wheels of change that brought us to the amazing world of culture, art, science, technology, and plenty in which we live today. But at the end of the day, with all our accomplishments, we are still biological organisms—and the bodies we inhabit haven't changed much in 150,000 years.

LIQUID DIET

Although people got some liquid from food, until the advent of agriculture twelve thousand years ago, the only drinks that passed our ancestors' lips were most likely water and, as infants, breast milk. Raising livestock led to the introduction of milk. Five thousand years later, Sumerians brewed the first beer, and wine production began in Central Asia. Coffee and tea followed two to three thousand years ago. But it wasn't until a bumper crop of Florida oranges were damaged by frost in the 1950s that juice became a widely marketed consumer product and our days began with sunshine.

The Land of Plenty

Our ability to preserve, store, and transport food increased over the years; giant leaps were made thanks to the Industrial Revolution. Our food supply became less cyclical and much more readily available. As a result, over the last 150 years, our diet underwent a radical and relatively abrupt set of changes that affected everything from the food we eat to the soil we grow it in.

There is a reason why Americans grow what we grow and eat what we eat, and it's because of how we grew as a nation. In the nineteenth century, as the East Coast cities swelled, all eyes turned toward the vast, unsettled West. The federal government recognized its chance to expand the Union and simultaneously to put millions of acres into production and feed the teeming urban centers. In 1862, President Lincoln signed into law the Homestead Act, which encouraged thousands of future farmers to head west, stake a claim on a piece of land, put down roots, and start farming for the nation. For their families, these pioneers tended gardens and orchards full of produce, which they consumed at its peak and preserved for the winter. However, without a modern, climate-controlled transportation system to ship their surplus commercial crops back to the eastern seaboard, their safest bet was to plant vast fields of grains, which could be dried, stored, and transported over long distances without spoiling. This was the birth of the modern American diet, centered on corn and wheat. Our larders were full, our sideboards bursting: It was a land of plenty.

With the amazing fortune of this incredibly fertile farmland, these Great Plains settlers produced the greatest abundance of food the world had ever seen. The nation built a vast railway network that ensured a constant supply of food to every corner of the expanding country, and the future was bright. We were happy. We were full. And over time our bellies grew.

The Modern (Processed) World

Today, because the intersection of our hugely productive agricultural system with consumer demand enables an efficient food industry, we live in an age of unprecedented abundance and convenience when it comes to food. Affordable food is now widely available, thanks to a powerful combination of fertilizers, pesticides, crop insurance, agricultural research, and federal subsidies to the farmers who grow commodity crops like wheat, corn, and soy.

In the first half of the twentieth century, as our factories grew, so did our farms. Mechanization took over much of the labor, and we no longer needed 50 percent of our workforce to work the land. As farm boys went to work in factories, and families moved to the cities and then to suburbs, Americans bought most of their food instead of producing it themselves. The government became concerned with stabilizing the production of food to guarantee a secure, steady, and cheap supply. By the 1950s, American farms were feeding the world. Small farms folded and larger ones consolidated until, by the 1980s, a handful of corporations were responsible for food production. And the few crops they were mainly interested in planting were corn, wheat, and soy (when scientists finally figured out how to extract and process its oil).

In the decades after World War II, women entered the workforce in larger numbers, an ever-increasing number of households had two working parents, and our suburbs spawned exurbs. Time became Americans' most precious commodity, and industry responded with more convenience products. The busier we got, the more important quick and easy food became. Eating out became the norm: The neighborhood diner begat Howard Johnson's begat the Olive Garden. Cooking became a lost art: The chicken in every pot became the nuggets in every microwave.

The staple grains that could be broken down—corn, wheat, soy, and rice—became America's new cash crops, and literally edged fruits and vegetables off the farm and off our plates. Today, more than two-thirds of the calories we consume come from those four crops. On average, Americans consume 1,670 calories from them every day. Over the last twenty years, the percentage of American adults who eat the recommended amount of fruits and vegetables a day dropped from 42 percent to 26 percent. Even more shocking? One-fourth of all vegetables consumed in the United States are eaten in the form of french fries or potato chips.

As our supply of corn and soy began to exceed even our capacity to eat it, agribusinesses looked for a new market. They found it in chickens, cows, and pigs. Twenty-five to fifty percent of the corn grown today is used to fatten our livestock. Cheap, subsidized corn and soy have turned our animal pastures into feedlots. These transformations in the meat, poultry, and dairy industries also changed our daily menus, as they made animal foods more affordable. This is likely one reason that Americans now consume close to two hundred pounds of meat and chicken per capita every year, fifty pounds more than we did fifty years ago.

When the raw materials are so inexpensive—far less costly than labor, rent, or advertising—manufacturers and restaurants are able to employ one of the most powerful marketing tactics: offering customers more value for their money. Portions today are two to five times larger than they used to be. We imagine that few restaurants have lost money on an all-you-can-eat buffet because, in today's world, the food is the cheapest cost of doing business.

PORTION DISTORTION

Average serving sizes have increased more than you might think. While our bagels today are as big as the plate they're served on, they used to fit in the palm of your hand. And keep in mind, the sizes available twenty years ago were usually the only option.

FOOD	20 YEARS AGO	TODAY
Cup of coffee	8 ounces: 45 calories	16 ounces: 350 calories
Bagel, plain	3-inch diameter: 140 calories	6-inch diameter: 350 calories
Blueberry muffin	1.5 ounces: 210 calories	5 ounces: 500 calories
Chicken Caesar salad with dressing	1½ cups: 390 calories	3 cups: 790 calories
Soda	6.5-ounce bottle: 85 calories	20-ounce bottle: 250 calories
French fries	2.4-ounce bag: 210 calories	6.9-ounce "large" bag: 610 calories

The Mismatch Between Our Bodies and Our World

We love the food we eat, and for the first time in human history most of us in the United States have more than enough of it—and that's a good thing. The problem, though, is that we evolved to expect a world where food was hard to find and where we had to work hard for it. Since we now find food at every turn, we eat far too much of it, without having to move any muscle but our jaws.

Sir Peter Gluckman and Mark Hanson characterized this conundrum in their book *Mismatch: Why Our World No Longer Fits Our Bodies*. As Gluckman puts it, "Our bodies were designed for one world, but we're living in a very different world"—one with far too much food and an excess of automation.

Rather than a lack of willpower or laziness, it is this inherent mismatch that has tipped the scales.

5

The Food We Eat

We all know that if you eat more and don't increase your activity level you will gain weight. And there's no denying that we're eating more. Our body is a complex system that strives to achieve a balance between how much energy we consume and how much we expend. Ingesting more than we need throws the delicate system off balance and creates a surplus. Where does that surplus end up? Your fat cells.

It doesn't matter where those excess calories come from—Big Macs, ice cream, Slurpees, or salad—if you take in too many calories, your body will store the extra as fat.

And we're consuming 31 percent more calories than we did forty years ago. In just the last twenty-five years, American adults have added 300 extra calories to their day; children have added an additional 200 calories. A small part of that is required to maintain our higher average weight, but the bulk of it is contributing instead to our national weight gain.

We snack so often now, and on so much food when we do, that snacks add up to a fourth or fifth meal every day. It's even worse for our kids. In 1980, children ate just one snack a day. Today they have an average of three, but one in five school-age children eats up to six snacks.

The fact that we are eating more is made worse by what our modern world serves up as food. If we were getting the extra three hundred calories from a single avocado, packed with vitamins, antioxidants, and omega-3 fatty acids, we would still be gaining weight, but eating those three hundred calories in the form of guacamole-flavored tortilla chips is probably adding insult to injury.

Are All Calories Created Equal?

Scientifically speaking, a *calorie* is by definition a measurement of the energy your body extracts from food. It's nothing else—not a measurement of weight, volume, or the complete story of how your body processes what you eat. That can make it tricky to determine if what you're eating is healthy based on calorie count alone.

There may be differences in how satisfying or filling a gram of protein is as compared with a gram of carbohydrate, but in terms of the energy your body extracts from food, a calorie is a calorie. It doesn't matter if you eat 1 calorie of lettuce or 1 calorie of cheesecake, your body will still extract 4.2 kilojoules of energy from it.

However, the calories are only one component of what we eat—the energy component. Foods contain more than just energy. They also provide us with vitamins, minerals (including sodium in the form of salt), fatty acids, amino acids, and fiber.

Your body doesn't process all these components in the same way. For instance, a saturated fatty acid (the bad kind, like the white marbling in a prime cut of beef) and a monounsaturated fatty acid (the good kind, like olive oil) will each do different things to the body's ability to make cholesterol: One harms it; one helps it. That can, in turn, influence disease development. So while your body deals with the energy of each calorie practically identically, the various components of a food act in different ways in the body.

If you're doing a diet reality check, the most important question to ask yourself is this: How many calories are you eating and drinking? If the number is too high, the best way to figure out what to retain and what to scrap is to take a good hard look at where those calories are coming from.

EMPTY CALORIES STILL COUNT

Sometimes food is referred to as having *empty calories*, but that doesn't mean they don't count. The calories will still be used for energy or stored as fat like any other calorie. They are only "empty" because energy is the only benefit they provide; they lack the other nutrients in healthier foods.

Fat in Your Food

One reason fat comes up so often in conversations about what not to eat is because it's the most calorie-dense macronutrient. Each gram of fat contains 9 calories, as opposed to the 4 calories per gram of protein or carbohydrate. Fat packs a lot of calories into a small space. It's the reason why a Caesar salad with dressing can have as many calories as a cheeseburger. Those aren't coming from the lettuce. But fat's not all bad. In fact, it's essential. And it's recommended that adults get between 20 and 35 percent of their daily calories from it.

From a dietary perspective, we are interested in three main kinds of edible fat, or technically, fatty acids: unsaturated, saturated, and trans fats, which are actually a subtype of unsaturated fat but act more like saturated fat.

Unsaturated Fats

Unsaturated fats are found naturally in plants and fish. They may help lower your blood's cholesterol levels, reduce the risk of cardiovascular disease, and increase insulin sensitivity—a good thing. There are two good kinds of unsaturated fats: monounsaturated and polyunsaturated. Omega-3 fatty acids—a type of polyunsaturated fat—have gotten a lot of attention lately because of their possible health-promoting benefits. Because the algae in the ocean's food chain contains omega-3s, as does the grass that constitutes the natural diet of cattle and chickens, when we eat pastured meat and wild cold-water fish (or fish oil), they are generally good sources of omega-3s. Because omega-3s have been shown to promote the health of the cell walls in our arteries, nervous systems, and brains, experts encourage us to eat foods containing them, like certain fish, and food manufacturers have started supplementing other foods with them.

Saturated Fats

Saturated fats come mostly from animal products, including meat, dairy, and egg yolks. Saturated fats may raise the levels of the harmful LDL cholesterol in your blood, but they might also slightly boost your helpful HDL cholesterol. Too much saturated fat may increase your risk of cardiovascular disease, while also adding unnecessary calories to your diet.

Our bodies make saturated fats, so they are not essential in our diet, and you should watch the amount you consume. Generally less than 10 percent of calories should come from saturated fatty acids. Less than 7 percent would be even better.

Trans Fats

Trans fats are also not essential in our diets and occur in nature in some animal products. But most trans fats are also industrially produced. To make them, food scientists use a combination of heat, hydrogen, and other chemicals to transform healthy unsaturated fats—mostly vegetable oils—into hydrogenated fats, which make for a more shelf-stable product with favorable cooking properties. If chemists take the oil through the entire process of hydrogenation, they end up with a saturated fat. But if they stop partway through, "partially hydrogenating" it, they can turn the oil into a solid that will last a very long time, is easy to ship, and is ideal for frying foods. When McDonald's and other fast-food restaurants stopped frying potatoes in beef fat, trans fats took over. The problem is that, when we consume these factory-modified partially hydrogenated fats, we suffer metabolic consequences. According to a 2002 IOM report, trans fats "provide no known benefit to human health" and can be harmful. Consuming trans fats has been shown not only to increase your bad cholesterol but also to decrease your good cholesterol.

Because trans fats are such a double whammy for our metabolism, we should avoid them. Fortunately, since 2006, the government has required that they be listed on all nutrition labels. If they constitute any part of a product you're thinking of buying, put the box down and back away. It's a good idea to check some products, like margarine, buttery spreads, vegetable shortening, microwave popcorn, pancake mix, and boxed cake mix especially closely, because almost all of them contain trans fats. And it's not just labels you need to read. Trans fats' properties are so appealing to manufacturers that many prepared foods, especially baked goods, and much of the fried food in chain restaurants, still contain them and are best avoided.

The official Dietary Guidelines for Americans recommend keeping trans fat intake as low as possible, but many Americans eat some industrially produced trans fats without being aware of it. Manufacturers can claim that a product contains "0 grams of trans fats" on the nutrition facts panel even if the product contains up to .5 grams of trans fats per serving. Always check the list of ingredients to see if the product contains any "partially hydrogenated" oil—such as corn, soy, or safflower—an indication that industrially produced trans fats are present. Your best defense against artificial trans fats is to buy, cook, and eat whole foods whenever possible.

FAT-BURNING FOODS: FACT AND FICTION

It sounds like a miracle—eat yourself thin!—but sadly there is no such thing as a "fat-burning food." The phrase is usually used as a ploy to get you interested in following a new diet plan. If the people using that claim go on to explain that certain foods, like those high in fiber, can help you feel full and eat less, thereby curbing an increase in caloric intake that could lead to weight gain, then they're correct. But if they claim that a specific food, like grapefruit or cabbage soup, will actually burn fat, they are spreading misinformation.

The only real way to burn fat is some combination of eating fewer calories than your body needs and increasing your activity level. When your body doesn't meet its daily energy needs from your food, or when you expend more energy than you take in, it will be forced to raid your fat stores. Your fat cells will shrink, as will your waistline. What should make you happier is that a smaller waist is a measure of better health, but there's no denying it can feel good to slip into smaller clothes, too.

The Problem with Refined Grains

To make refined flour, the bran and the germ are removed from the wheat kernel, which removes much of its dietary fiber and other nutrients, like vitamins. Some of the nutrients are then added back in, to "enrich" the flour, but the fiber is not. The result is flour that takes a lot longer to spoil, keeps well on the shelf, and has different effects on our bodies than the original whole grain. When white flour was invented during the Industrial Revolution, it was hailed as a solution for feeding the hungry masses. But, for most of us in the United States today, whole grains are a better bet for our health.

When we eat whole grains, much of the fiber passes through our body as what our grandmothers might have called "roughage." This gives us a sense of fullness and has other health benefits. When a factory removes the fiber for us, it results in a powder, such as white flour, that is an easy-to-digest starch that breaks down into glucose quickly. The flood of glucose in the bloodstream causes insulin levels to spike because one of insulin's jobs is to move glucose from the blood into the cells to provide them with energy, after which blood sugar levels go down, causing hunger and making you think you need to eat again.

Little Changes = Big Results

There's a reason you hear a lot about whole grains. If they're truly whole, they're good for you. Compared to refined grains, they take more time to digest, keep you full longer, and come jam-packed with naturally occurring vitamins and minerals, so make them an important part of your diet. The problem with "whole" is that it's an unregulated word. Food manufacturers can make all sorts of claims about whole-grain content even when they add an insignificant amount of fiber back into their enriched pastas, breads, and cereals. To ensure that you're buying 100 percent whole grain products, look for labels that say "100% whole wheat," for example, and skip products that use the words "enriched" or "refined" to describe the grains in the ingredient list. Keep in mind that you still have to pay attention to portion size, even with brown rice and steel-cut oats.

Sweet Loving

There's a reason almost everyone has a sweet tooth, and that's because our brain, the ultimate boss of our bodies, requires a steady supply of glucose. When it comes to sugar, we're no different from many other species—we love it. Nothing says more about how pleasurable it is than the sight of lab rats enduring the jolts of an electric shock in order to obtain one more sip of sugar water. Like all those other things that are essential to survival, nature's sugar is intensely pleasurable for us.

As neuroscientist Nora Volkow explains, pleasure and learning are inextricably linked. If you don't believe her, try going to a park on a summer day and watch what happens when the ice cream truck pulls up. Scientists who study these kinds of things believe that this Pavlovian reaction has its roots in the time of our hunter-gatherer ancestors. They theorize that when our ancestors came across the rare piece of ripe, juicy fruit, or discovered a beehive, they needed to remember where it was in order to survive. What's the best way to make a memory stick and encourage us to repeat the experience? Make it as enjoyable as possible. (For more on this, see chapter 7, "Know Thy Brain.")

SUGAR BABY

The work of Dr. Julie Mennella, a taste researcher at the Monell Chemical Senses Center in Philadelphia, shows that infants love the taste of sugar from the moment they're born. It's not clear whether babies love sugar because breast milk is sweet, or if breast milk evolved to be sweet so that infants would nurse unprompted, but either way, one thing is clear: Sugar is every baby's favorite flavor.

For that reason, the consumption of a variety of foods that are nutrient-rich, rather than sugar-rich, should be encouraged. To introduce foods high in added sugars into the diet too early sets children up for a lifetime of sugar cravings without the learned love of other flavors that comes with a healthy, balanced diet.

The Complexities of Carbohydrates

The carbohydrates we eat, whether starches or sugars, are chains of carbon, oxygen, and hydrogen that serve as an energy source for the body. Starches—also known as complex carbohydrates—are long chains of carbohydrate molecules, found in the vegetables we eat, the potatoes we mash, the rice we boil, and the grains we turn into flour for making pasta, bread, and cookies. In order for them to fuel the body's cells, they need to be broken down into simple carbohydrates, whether by our own digestion or in a factory when they're refined. Sugars—simple carbohydrates—are disaccharides, meaning the chains are only two units long.

The substance we most commonly think of as table sugar, the white granules that we add to our coffee and that put the frost in Frosted Flakes, is known scientifically as sucrose. Sucrose is derived from sugar cane or sugar beets and is made up of one molecule of glucose and one molecule of fructose. The first natural source of such concentrated sweetness our ancestors encountered was probably honey. Every beehive is a miniature sugar refinery, where worker bees transform flower nectar into a substance that is chemically similar to table sugar.

There's lots of confusing talk about high-fructose corn syrup, which is actually a bit of a misnomer. The important thing to understand is that high-fructose corn syrup, chemically derived from corn, is also a combination of glucose and fructose, though not always in a 50/50 ratio.

Some types of high-fructose corn syrup have more than 50 percent fructose and some have a bit less, but high-fructose corn syrup earned its name simply because it contains more fructose than plain old corn syrup.

A SIMPLE SUGAR PRIMER

Whether we consume carbohydrates in complex or simple form, the body metabolizes them into individual sugar molecules, known as monosaccharides. Here's a summary of how they break down:

Glucose

The critical energy source required by all our cells, especially those that make up our brains, glucose occurs naturally in carbohydrates but must be broken down from longer chains by our digestive system before we can use it. Once carbohydrates are fully broken down, glucose then enters the bloodstream, and insulin transports it to all the cells of the body to meet our immediate energy needs. If excess glucose remains after these needs have been met, it is stored in the liver and muscles in the form of glycogen, which gives us quick and easy access to energy to sustain us overnight and between meals. Any excess glucose that's still coursing through our blood after glycogen formation is converted into fat and stored.

Fructose

Also known as "fruit sugar" because it's found in fruit, fructose is much sweeter than glucose, and occurs in much smaller amounts in food naturally. Dr. Robert Lustig, a neuroendocrinologist at the University of California–San Francisco (UCSF), believes that because we rarely encountered fructose in such high concentrations in the course of our evolution, the body did not develop a system to harness its energy efficiently. The excess fructose we now consume due to all the added sugars in our diet is converted by the liver into fat and stored there. If there is enough excess table sugar or high-fructose corn syrup in our sodas and other sweetened processed foods, the fat that accumulates in our liver can overtake it, making them primary contributors to nonalcoholic fatty liver disease.

High-Fructose Corn Syrup

High-fructose corn syrup is a man-made blend of purified sugars derived from corn, invented in the 1970s in Japan. It is very similar to table sugar, in that it contains roughly equal proportions of glucose and fructose. The crucial thing to remember, whenever you hear the word fructose, is that too much of it is undesirable no matter the source—high-fructose corn syrup, table sugar, honey, or agave nectar, which range from 56 percent to a whopping 92 percent fructose.

How Much Sugar Are We Adding?

One of the most momentous changes in the American diet since 1909—when the U.S. Department of Agriculture (USDA) first began keeping track—has been the increase in the percentage of calories coming from sugars that are added to foods. Sugars occur naturally in small amounts in many foods—like apples and milk—and are also added to foods. Added sugars have many names, such as white sugar, brown sugar, turbinado sugar, corn syrup, corn syrup solids, high-fructose corn syrup, maltose syrup, maple syrup, pancake syrup, fructose sweetener, liquid fructose, honey, molasses, anhydrous dextrose, and crystalline dextrose. Add them all together and we are consuming more added sugars, and with them more calories.

According to the USDA, the average American consumes 156 pounds of added sugars every year. That's the equivalent of two and a half five-pound bags of sugar a month per person, poured over (or hiding inside) your food.

The World Health Organization released guidelines in 2003 recommending we get no more than 10 percent of our daily calories from added sugars. On a 2,000-calorie-a-day diet, that would mean 200 calories, or about twelve teaspoons. With almost fourteen teaspoons of sugar sloshing around inside, a twenty-ounce bottle of non-diet soda would put you over your limit.

A recent study of teens around the country found they are consuming more than double that recommended amount of sugar. The average teen reported consuming 480 calories a day from added sugars, which amounted to 21 percent of their calorie intake.

How Added Sugars Can Make You Fat

Obviously, added sugars give our bodies more sugar than they're used to or need.

Mountains of added sugars mean the human metabolism now has to contend with more simple carbohydrates than it has ever encountered before. In the natural world, sugar is a rare treasure, typically encountered seasonally in ripe fruit, packaged in a whole food full of fiber and valuable micronutrients. When it came in the form of honey, we had to brave a swarm of angry bees to obtain it.

Our overconsumption of all types of sugar may be overwhelming our bodies' well-calibrated systems. The body knows glucose only as a precious raw material, so it absorbs as much as it can into the blood.

Like too much of anything, too much sugar in the blood is toxic, so insulin saves us from hyperglycemia (high blood sugar) by rapidly transforming excess glucose into fat.

How Liquid Calories Can Make You Fat

Thanks to the relatively recent invention of soda, sweetened tea, juice, vitamin waters, energy drinks, and specialty coffee drinks, we're drinking a lot of calories. Calories consumed from sweetened beverages increased 135 percent from 1977 to 2001. That's a lot of extra calories for our bodies to handle.

Until beer and wine were invented, our early ancestors likely drank only two things: breast milk and water. Breast milk fulfilled almost all of the body's nutritional requirements in infancy. Water didn't. Drinking water is absolutely essential to survival, but it doesn't override the need for food, for good reason. Imagine what would have happened to our hunter-gatherer forebears if their hunger were sated by drinking water. They wouldn't feel the need to forage for food and wouldn't store enough essential body fat for times of famine. If water consumption alleviated our hunger pangs we might not have survived as a species.

There is some evidence suggesting that, regardless of how many calories are in our drinks, the act of drinking probably doesn't curb our appetite as much as eating food does. Ideally, we should get very few of our calories from beverages, and, when we do, we should cut the same number of calories from our food intake. But we usually don't, because our brain often tells us we're still hungry. In the face of our increased consumption of caloric beverages, our body's difficulty with "counting" those calories can lead to excess caloric intake, which leads to—you guessed it—fat storage.

Little Changes = **Big Results**

At coffee shops and juice stands, **order the smallest size drink possible,** such as the child-size, if available. Specify nonfat milk, and skip the whipped cream. The menu board might say the smallest size is a twelve-ounce "tall," but ask that your drink be poured into an eight-ounce "short" cup. You'll shave off over 30 percent of the calories, no matter what you order.

6

Know Thy Body

same foundation of evidence as everything you'll know by the time you get to the end of this book.

Elana keeps careful account of the calories she consumes and knows that, with the number of calories she's decided to take in, she needs to walk six miles a day to keep the weight off. She now knows her body so well that if she decides to indulge in ice cream one night, she will walk an extra mile the next morning. Surprised that she can have her cake and walk it off, too? As Elana puts it, "A diet has an end point. But my new way of life is a process. This is something I'm going to be doing my entire life, and I'm not willing to live my life deprived."

Her walking buddy, Rhonda, who at four feet ten inches has also lost more than a hundred pounds, says, "I didn't gain weight overnight, and I'm not going to lose the weight overnight. It's a journey."

Both of them know enough about success and failure in life and weight loss that they never want to fail again. Their secret to success? They have learned to make their goals small enough that they can be 100 percent achievable.

"I understand that it's calories in, calories out," Elana says. "It's just math. And now I understand how much work it takes to make it all add up. I'm just an ordinary person who does a whole bunch of very tiny ordinary things that together are extraordinary. And it's so worth it."

Your body is in balance when you're consuming the same amount of energy (calories) per day as you are burning (expending). Think of a scale: On one side is the amount of calories you take in; on the other side is the number of calories you expend. If both sides are even, you're in balance.

A common misconception is that overweight people are out of balance because they are eating too much. If their weight is stable, they are actually in balance: They're eating the amount of food they need to stay at their current weight.

When we eat more calories than we burn, we gain weight. To lose weight, we need to do the opposite: Take in fewer calories than we're burning. Or, to think of it the other way, burn more calories than we are taking in. Either way—exercising more or eating less—tips the balance in a healthier direction.

If you need to lose weight, the easiest way to go about it is by staying within a certain calorie budget—less than what your body needs to maintain its current weight, but still enough to allow proper functioning and to minimize hunger pangs. Adding more physical activity into your life is a good way to increase that budget: The more you move, the more you'll be able to eat, but you still have to expend more calories than you consume. When you eventually reach your healthy weight, you will need to continue balancing calories in with calories out to maintain it. People who have lost significant amounts of weight, like Elana, will likely end up with a smaller calorie budget than they're used to and need to monitor it carefully in order to maintain their new, lower weight.

Little Changes = Big Results

Set yourself a calorie budget—and stick to it!

Start by keeping track of every morsel and sip that enters your mouth and recording it in a calorie counter online or on your smartphone—a good, old-fashioned journal works, too. After a while, you'll have a vivid picture of what you are eating and drinking day in and day out. When you consider your total intake, you can begin to figure out how much you need to cut back and where might be a good place to begin cutting. If the cuts you have to make seem too drastic, add physical activity to offset the need to reduce your intake so much.

Weight Regulations

For a long time, it was believed that excess weight was a direct result of a person's poor choices and lack of willpower. If someone didn't want to be overweight, they should simply eat less.

Some scientists weren't convinced the answer was so simple, however. They felt there must be more mechanisms controlling our weight than just the conscious decision to raise fork to mouth. After decades of research, they discovered that body weight is a tightly regulated system of complex metabolic reactions, managed by the body just like blood pressure or blood sugar. To a great extent, we no more choose to eat than we choose to fall asleep. There are basic, biological regulatory systems that operate below our conscious awareness. Knowing more about the internal systems that drive you to seek food and store excess calories as fat can help you better understand, and override, some of your body's powerful, innate signals.

Feed Me

There are two primary hormones that tell your body when it's running on empty: leptin and ghrelin.

Leptin is a hormone produced in fat cells and released into the bloodstream when food is consumed. It's in constant communication with our brains, reporting on the adequacy of our fat stores. According to Dr. Rudy Leibel, one of the scientists who discovered leptin and its role in regulating body weight, the more fat cells you have, and the fuller they are, the more leptin you have in circulation. When leptin reaches the brain, it is taken up by a region called the hypothalamus—the brain's center for controlling hunger. Like a thermostat in your home, always set to a particular temperature and ready to send a signal to fire up the furnace if it senses the temperature has dropped, the hypothalamus senses when leptin levels have dropped below normal, and sends its own signals to the rest of the brain, motivating all sorts of food-seeking behavior in an attempt to increase our fat levels, which in turn restores the leptin levels. This system was fine-tuned over the course of millions of years of food scarcity, as a way of ensuring that we always had a little fat in our bellies to tide us over till the next kill or till we stumbled into the next bramble of ripe berries.

Lose a few pounds? No matter how heavy you are, a drop in leptin is a signal of scarcity, and your brain will do whatever it takes to protect you. The hypothalamus has no way of knowing how many extra pounds you're carrying, or that you've got a refrigerator full of food and a convenience store on the corner.

Ghrelin, the other hormone that sends signals to your brain when you need more fuel, is released by your stomach when it is empty. Ghrelin makes you feel hungry, reminding you to seek food. However, in our current world of excess, we no longer need to jump every time our stomach rumbles. In many cases, we shouldn't.

Set Point

If your weight is currently stable, regardless of whether you're overweight or not, your leptin levels are normal. And your hypothalamus likes them that way. Your brain will defend that set point with everything it's got.

The discovery of leptin in 1994 by Dr. Rudy Leibel and others at Rockefeller University radically changed the way scientists think about the regulation of body weight. For the first time, it was established that weight is regulated at least in part hormonally, not entirely psychologically. This was proof that it's not only about personal choice and willpower. It's not just in our heads.

Subsequent studies have proved that leptin is involved in a phenomenon that scientists have noted for decades: When your weight increases, your set point rises along with it. The common belief that, when we lose weight our body fights to bring us back up to where we started, appears to be true. When our weight drops, leptin levels drop, and the brain dispatches signals to the body to try to protect us from the perceived threat of starvation.

Prior to the nineteenth century, our ancestors could barely even dream of a life where they didn't have to worry about going hungry. Now we're almost infinitely more likely to keel over from a heart attack than starve to death. But the dozens of body–brain connections that developed over the millennia to protect our fat stores, defend our set point, and ensure that we don't waste away have no equivalent for saving us from the devastating health effects of carrying too much weight.

Why would they? Not only did we rarely have the opportunity over the course of our evolution to become fat, but the health effects of excess weight take decades to develop, and we wouldn't have lived long enough to experience them anyway because accidents, infectious diseases, and the rigors of childbirth led to relatively early deaths for most of our ancestors. So nature favored those of us who could put on weight because storing excess fat gave us a survival advantage. As a result, there is not a single system in the human body that can break the bad news to our brains that we've packed on too many pounds, because only our minds perceive that as bad news.

The brain fails to comprehend our modern predicament. That lack of recognition means that, while our set point climbs higher as we gain weight, it can probably not be reset lower. When we lose weight—however necessary it might be for our health and happiness—our internal thermostat sounds an alarm, mobilizing all its forces and entering full-on famine-protection mode to thwart our best-intentioned efforts. If a morbidly obese man begins to shed excess pounds, his brain will still detect a drop in leptin, even though he might have billions of extra fat cells still in reserve. His brain will believe that he's starving, bringing on the hunger pangs and focusing his thoughts on food.

AN INCONVENIENT TRUTH

Your journey to become healthier and slimmer is no small feat. And when you start shedding those love handles, you may experience moments when your body and brain can feel like your worst enemies. In 1944, Ancel Keys, a researcher well known for developing rations for combat troops (K-rations), performed the groundbreaking Minnesota Starvation Experiment. This yearlong study, carried out during World War II on young, healthy, conscientious objectors, analyzed the physiological and psychological effects of prolonged diet restrictions. What did he discover? Over a six-month period, these hale and hearty men lost 25 percent of their body weight, but, in a surprise to Keys and to the men themselves, it was extremely hard for them to stick to their diets. Most of them became obsessed with food, often binge-eating. It didn't stop with daydreams of mashed potatoes and buttered corn or nighttime raids on the commissary. Subjects also battled depression, social withdrawal, low libido, and even, in the most extreme case, self-mutilation.

But anyone who's ever tried to lose weight is probably not too surprised to hear this. Losing weight can be a miserable experience.

Till Death Do Us Part

Here is where we have to break some bad news to you: Even if you succeed at getting back down to a healthy weight, your body won't get on board and embrace it. Your brain will not believe your leptin levels are normal. And it will be difficult for your body to accept your new weight as its status quo. The research of Dr. Leibel and his colleague, Dr. Michael Rosenbaum, shows that even after ten years of successfully maintaining a significant weight loss, the body doesn't readjust. Your brain still thinks you're in a state of deprivation, and it manipulates your body in ways you don't even notice: You're hungrier, less easily satisfied, and more frequently tempted by sweet and fatty foods; you are less inclined to exercise, an effort by your body to conserve what fat stores it still detects; you even process food more efficiently, getting more miles per gallon out of what you eat and squirreling calories away in your hips, thighs, or belly.

Take as an example a forty-year-old woman who weighs two hundred pounds. Let's call her Ellen. Ellen never struggled with her weight as a teen or in her twenties, but after two pregnancies, she just couldn't lose the weight. But she wants to change, and she does. Ellen worked hard over the course of a year and reached her goal of losing 20 percent of her body weight. She lost forty pounds and now weighs 160. But her set point hasn't changed. She now requires 20 percent fewer calories than another 160-pound woman who has never been overweight.

Ellen happens to have a best friend—we'll call her Kate—who fits that bill exactly. The two of them do everything together, including walking half an hour every day and playing tennis on the weekends. They think of themselves as practically sisters, similar in almost every way. But when it comes to leptin and the set point, they will always be different. Ellen understands that when they go out to dinner (and all the rest of the time), she needs to consume 20 percent fewer calories than Kate does in order to maintain her new, trim figure. It's not fair, but it's the only way she'll keep the weight off.

A LITTLE BIT OF LEPTIN

As much as this chapter might have you hoping for a magic pill that would make maintaining weight loss a less daunting proposition, that prospect is still decades in the future, if it's possible at all. One of the brightest spots on the horizon, though, comes from new, groundbreaking research on leptin.

One of the first things that scientists tried after the discovery of leptin was injecting it into subjects to see if it helped them lose weight. Sadly, it made no difference. However, in a groundbreaking study of obese people who were carefully brought down to a reduced weight, Drs. Leibel and Rosenbaum of Columbia University's New York Obesity Research Center showed that injecting small amounts of leptin—just enough to replace the leptin they had lost when they shrank their fat cells by losing weight—could make it easier to keep weight off. These "replacement levels" of leptin may work to trick your brain into believing you're still fat, preventing it from unleashing its anti-starvation defense forces and letting you live at a healthier weight without suffering the metabolic changes and cravings that normally come along with leptin deprivation.

It will take a lot more time, money, and research before leptin could leap from the lab to the prescription pad, but it's encouraging to know that researchers are finding optimism in this area of drug development that has posed such a challenge.

Every single person who's ever lost weight—whether they needed to or not, whether they were fitting into a wedding gown, slimming down for the summer, or responding to their doctor telling them they had to lose a few pounds—has experienced this unfortunate condition. We know this is a bitter pill to swallow, and we're not going to sugar-coat it for you. As hard as it is to lose weight, it's more difficult to keep it off.

But as Elana, our video editor from New York, and thousands of others like her will tell you, there are ways of managing a life of leptin deprivation. And the most powerful tool we have to offer you is knowledge: knowledge about the systems within your body that fight against you, the forces in our modern world that you are up against, and the little things that you can do to fight back. And the promise, coming from Elana, that it's worth it.

7

Know Thy Brain

It's probably clear by now that little happens in the body without the brain having a say. In most cases, the brain monitors, controls, and influences everything.

Our Big, Fat Brain

Compared to the rest of the natural world, healthy human babies are born fat; the only other mammal that delivers chubbier offspring is the hooded seal (because they swim in that really cold water). Why do our babies need so much fat from birth? Because they need to develop big brains between the time they're born and the time they hit puberty. Infants can't be born with the big brains they'll eventually develop, because their heads would be too large to fit through the birth canal, posing a threat to both mother and infant during labor. When our distant ancestors began to leave the trees behind and walk upright, the human pelvis narrowed, which in turn narrowed the birth canal and forced our offspring to undergo much of their brain development outside the womb.

Our adorably chubby babies are born complete with extra fat reserves in case they enter into a world of scarcity, but in most cases, they find abundant supplies of fat in the form of breast milk.

All milk is not the same; each animal makes a special blend of milk to ensure the health of its young. One of the things that makes human breast milk so perfect for our babies is the amount and types of fat in it. Breast milk contains a wide variety of fatty acids that are crucial for a baby's optimal brain development. If you are a nursing mother, the best way to ensure your breast milk is replete with all the fats, vitamins, and minerals your baby needs is for you to consume a nutrient-rich diet. You may be what you eat, but your baby's brain is, too!

BREAST-FEEDING REDUCES OBESITY RISK

Dr. Matt Gillman, a researcher at Harvard Medical School, and his colleagues conducted a study, which found that breast-fed babies had a 20 percent lower risk of being overweight as preteens and teenagers when compared to formula-fed infants. They believe breast milk might give babies an early "metabolic programming" that leads to less fat accumulation in later years. Gillman also credits how breast-feeding allows the baby to have more control over how much he or she eats. A satisfied infant will pull away from the breast, whereas bottle-feeding parents might feel their baby is only full and properly fed when the bottle is empty. The opportunity breast-fed infants have to develop an innate sense of when they are full may help protect them against obesity later in life.

Hedonism 101

As discussed in chapter 5, pleasure and learning go hand in hand. When we experience something pleasurable, we remember it. The pleasure is something worth repeating.

Imagine one of our early ancestors walking in the woods with her young son. She finds an apple and gives it to him. He eats it; it's sweet and delicious. The child learns to connect everything about that experience with the pleasure he derived from the apple. The reason why pleasure and learning are inextricably bound is because the chemicals released in the brain to signify pleasure are the same neurotransmitters the brain uses to cement a memory. This connection between pleasure and memory formation is fundamental to the survival of any species. When scientists trying to understand the mechanisms that underlie this reward system sever it in lab animals, the animals experience no pleasure from food, stop seeking it, and die.

Our need for pleasure drives our survival instinct. In the case of the boy above, he will always associate red with ripeness, he will always see an apple tree as a source of delicious food, and he will always recognize one from across the forest. As he grows, he'll come across not just other apple trees, but pear trees, and peaches and plums, he'll gather all sorts of berries, and he'll learn to gather honey from a beehive. Each new experience will reinforce the previous ones, and as he continues to receive pleasure from the bounty that nature provides, he will learn to survive.

The brain's reward system is no less at play in our modern world. If anything, it's overwhelmed by our infinite food choices. Today, families don't come upon ripe apple trees as often as they do McDonald's, where children learn to associate the Golden Arches with pleasant memories of Happy Meals, playgrounds, and free toys, all designed to stimulate the release of pleasure chemicals in the brain. Think how strong those memories will be (or how strong your own are). That alone could be enough to keep you coming back for a Big Mac and a smile for the rest of your life.

Habit Forming

When we experience the pleasure of sweet, fatty food, our brains release dopamine and serotonin. If that food also contains chocolate, for example, endorphins are released as well. The food industry knows all about our pleasure pathways and, when it adds salt to fat and sugar, it creates maximally desirable foods. When we eat one of these "hyperpalatable" foods—a chocolate-covered pretzel is a classic example—fireworks go off inside us. Research has shown that consuming these kinds of foods soon becomes a habit.

How much of a habit? A study at the Scripps Research Institute found that rats that were overfed junk food adopted the same compulsive habits they'd exhibit in the case of drug addiction. The pleasure center of the brain gets overloaded and eventually crashes, leaving the rat scrambling to find more. Brain scans of people eating junk food light up in the same way as scans of drug addicts.

Dr. Gene-Jack Wang, a neuroscientist at Brookhaven National Laboratory, isn't surprised about the possible similarities between junk food consumption and drug use. "We make our food very similar to cocaine now," he says. "We purify [it]. Our ancestors ate whole grains, but we're eating white bread. American Indians ate corn; we eat corn syrup."*

Bring in the Top Executive

Now that you know there is a real but entirely subconscious power that pulls you toward unhealthy foods, what can you do about it? Understanding how your brain's reward system works can help you override it.

The part of the human brain associated with pleasure is among the most ancient parts of the brain—ours is almost identical to that of a mouse. But there's a much more recently evolved region of the brain called the prefrontal cortex, which is far more developed in humans than in mice, dogs, or even monkeys. The prefrontal cortex, most of which sits just behind your forehead, is the hub of the network that forms the executive center of your brain. This network is where decision-making happens. It's what we use to plan ahead, consider all our options, and control our impulses. The prefrontal cortex is also one of the last regions of the brain to finish developing. If you don't believe us, spend some time with anyone under the age of eighteen.

Your prefrontal cortex is your brain's CEO. If the rest of your brain has a hard time obeying company policy in the face of sweet temptations, it may be time to call in the big brass to get everyone else in line. According to neuroscientist Dr. Nora Volkow, the reason it's so hard for most of us to resist temptation is that we've never had to turn down food before. We have no automatic system to do this, so we must reason our way out of every bad decision. In our modern world, where tasty food is everywhere, our CEO is forced to work overtime to prevent us from eating all day long, and sometimes gives up. Often without us even being aware of it, our hand reaches back into the big bag of chips, and before we know it, we've eaten half of it.

PART III

‖‖‖‖‖‖‖‖‖‖‖‖‖‖‖‖‖‖‖‖‖‖‖‖‖‖‖‖

The Forces Working Against Us

Biologically, we're at odds with our modern world. As Michael Power and Jay Schulkin, the authors of *The Evolution of Obesity*, put it: "We evolved on the savannas of Africa, and we now live in Candyland."

As if that weren't bad enough, despite our best efforts to lose weight and be healthy—or to prevent weight gain in the first place—there are numerous outside influences that make it very difficult for us to make the changes we desire. This information isn't meant to scare or depress you; it's meant to empower you. To quote everyone from Thomas Hobbes to *Schoolhouse Rock*: "Knowledge is power." Unless we are aware of the secrets, tactics, and messages that subliminally target us and our children, we cannot begin to counteract them.

Who exactly are we up against? Welcome to the *World vs Us*.

8

Fast Food vs Us

L et's start with an easy one: One in four Americans visit a fast-food restaurant every single day. In 1970, Americans spent $6 billion on fast food. In 2006, we spent $142 billion.

What keeps us going back, even though we know eating too much of it is not good for us? Fast food serves up what we crave most—sugar, fat, and salt—and what we value most—squeezing more out of our food dollars. Sometimes they even add a little inexpensive novelty in the form of a tiny toy. And, let's not forget that it's the "fast" in fast food that gives us more time to do all the things we need to do in our time-limited, stressful lives.

The fast-food industry has made improvements in many areas: offering healthier options, like the apple slices McDonald's has added to Happy Meals, and higher quality ingredients. But "healthier" doesn't always mean healthy. And in terms of portion sizes, they are unintentionally endangering the lives of their customers.

Super Super Sizes

While the fast-food industry pulled back on giant sizes in 2004, following a public and government outcry, its concern for our nation's obesity problem seems to have been short-lived. In fact, they doubled down.

Rather than just offering their regular menu items in bigger buckets, restaurants created what is known in the industry as the oversize concept sandwich.

First came KFC's Double Down: bacon, cheese, and mayo-based sauce held not by bread, but by two fried chicken patties. Its success—in just two months, KFC sold 10 million of them—had fast-food chains scrambling to outdo each other. There were soon foot-long cheeseburgers, burgers served between two grilled cheese sandwiches, grilled cheese stuffed with mozzarella sticks, patty melts stuffed with macaroni and cheese, and perhaps the granddaddy of them all, Burger King's Pizza Burger, an almost ten-inch-diameter, 2,530-calorie monster. When *Time* magazine asked Brad Haley, vice president of marketing for CKE Restaurants, the parent company of Carl's Jr. and Hardee's, which sells the 1,120-calorie, 72-grams-of-fat Double Steakhouse Burger, to explain the megaburger trend, his response was simple and unapologetic: "This is what everyone in the industry is doing now."

RED AND YELLOW KILL A FELLOW

Fast-food restaurants start working on your resolve from fifty feet down the street. Their logos are almost all colored red and yellow for a reason—to lure you from afar. Interestingly enough, these are the colors that in nature signify ripeness: Bright red and yellow fruit stands out against a sea of green leaves, which lets us spot it from a distance. The color red is believed to increase blood pressure; yellow is a happy color, and the easiest to see in daylight. Together, they are purported to start your stomach rumbling.

Coincidence? Maybe not. Trust your instincts and drive away.

Fast-food restaurants are well aware that if they bundle individual items into combos with giant sizes, people will end up eating more and coming back for more.

A 2010 study published in the *Journal of Public Policy & Marketing* found that participants ordered smaller sizes when the only options were à la carte. When combos were available, customers overwhelmingly bought them, thinking they were getting a good deal. But in reality, unbeknownst to the consumers looking only to save money, they're getting more food. Most combo-size servings are larger than what people would order à la carte. Making it more expensive to buy smaller portions leads customers to eat a lot more calories than they bargained for.

Plus, the pleasure we derive from eating diminishes with each subsequent bite. Hand someone a small bag of fries, and by the time they dig out that last, salty, crunchy bit jammed into the corner of the greasy bag, they'll probably be just as satisfied as if you'd handed them a jumbo one.

Mark Hardison, vice president of El Pollo Loco, concedes that they considered doing away with combo meals as they were introducing healthier options, but guests "overwhelmingly" wanted the combos back. "As long as our guests are getting a good value out of that, we're happy to complete their meal. It makes business more economically viable and our business performance stronger when we do it that way."*

But if we really aren't asking for more food, just bigger savings, why give us more food then, essentially for free?

Little Changes = **Big Results**

You don't have to completely swear off fast food; just swear off its supersized combos and value menus, knowing they are traps for your biology and psychology. Yes, you might lose twenty cents ordering each item individually, but what you'll gain health-wise will more than make up for it. Resist the upsell, refuse the upgrade, and order the smallest size available. Choosing the small fries over the large at McDonald's could save you 270 calories and 14 grams of fat!

— 9 —

Restaurants vs Us

Americans have never thought more about food than we do today. From *Top Chef* fanatics, burger bloggers, and devotees of *Diners, Drive-ins and Dives* to foodies who rhapsodize about heirloom vegetables and homeowners who covet high-powered professional ranges, food has become a national obsession. But, all too often, we're obsessing over the wrong kind of food and, even when our food obsessions are virtuous, they don't usually manifest in our kitchens and on our plates. Face it. Americans just don't cook that much anymore.

We now get a third of our calories from eating out—almost double the amount from thirty years ago. Lisa Mancino, a food economist for the USDA, says that, for the average consumer, eating just one meal a week away from home can translate to two extra pounds of weight gain a year. Considering more than half of American adults eat out three or more times a week, and 12 percent eat out more than once a day, it's easy to see how restaurants have contributed to our national weight gain.

As former Food and Drug Administration (FDA), commissioner David Kessler describes in his book *The End of Overeating*, the layering of sugar and fat with a fair shake of salt—apple pie with ice cream is an example—goes a long way toward explaining why a night out can pack on so many more calories than a dinner at home.

Extreme Entrées

If we looked only at the supersized offerings of fast-food chains, we'd be missing a big part of the problem. Full-service restaurants also offer oversized and unhealthy menu items. While the most indulgent dishes used to weigh in at around 1,000 calories, many now offer more than your entire daily caloric allowance on a single plate. The Cheesecake Factory's Pasta Carbonara with Chicken boasts 2,500 calories and 85 grams of saturated fat. (That's 65 more grams of saturated fat than the FDA recommends for an entire day for a person consuming 2,000 calories a day!) Follow that dish with its Chocolate Tower Truffle Cake and you'll add another 1,670 calories—the equivalent of fourteen Hostess Ho Hos. One order of Outback Steakhouse Aussie Cheese Fries, complete with bacon and ranch dressing, clocks in at 2,900 calories and 182 grams of fat.

And don't be fooled by "healthier" options. Turkey burgers and fish tacos have to be better choices than a hamburger or burrito, right? Not always. Ruby Tuesday's Bella Turkey Burger has 1,145 calories and 71 grams of fat. Order On the Border's Dos XX Fish Tacos in fresh flour tortillas with rice and beans and you'll get 2,100 calories and 130 grams of fat. That's a lot of time on a treadmill—more than four hours of jogging.

Little Changes = **Big Results**

The restaurant industry knows that "healthy" has become a buzzword. And who doesn't want to be healthier? But just because the restaurant calls its turkey burger a "healthier" option—even if they've marked it on the menu with a little green leaf or other symbol—does *not* always mean that it's healthy.

It's up to you to ask yourself, "Healthier than what?" Ordering the turkey burger that they claim is "healthier" may be a good place to start, but ask them to hold the mayo or the cheese and to swap the fries for a salad (dressing on the side), or just leave the top of the bun behind before you sink your teeth into the burger.

Designed for Your Engorgement

Restaurants aren't only serving us bigger portions; cues to eat more are built into their designs. It's no accident that popular chain restaurants have loud music, blaring TVs, and dim lighting. That "atmosphere" is intended to prompt people to eat more and make it easy to do so. Restaurants like these are playing on those same instincts that drive us to overeat whenever we have the chance, but especially when we're stressed.

- **Loud music:** Can raise people's heart rate and cause them to eat faster. Eating too fast means you might keep eating right past when you're really full.
- **TVs:** Researchers found we eat 14 percent more when distracted by a TV. Some restaurants have added one in every corner.
- **Dim lights:** Keep us from clearly seeing what or how much we're eating.

SUCCESS STORIES

There are, however, ways to combat the noise and distractions that pervade not just restaurants, but so much of our lives as well. Dr. Elissa Epel, a research psychologist and the director of UCSF's Center for Obesity Assessment, Study & Treatment, has studied the effects of stress on eating behavior and obesity. Her research shows the value of adopting a more mindful approach to food.

Tom, a retired San Francisco police officer, was morbidly obese when he signed up for one of Dr. Epel's studies about a year ago. Before then, he says, "As a police officer, I worked irregular hours. I ate irregularly, too—a lot of fast food. Mindless eating would describe me very well. I would eat a sandwich in five bites. My mother died of heart disease at age fifty-seven. I'm fifty-six. And I got to a place where I almost thought, 'Well, she lived a good life.' I was pretty resigned to being the way I was."

But Dr. Epel's study taught Tom to take a more mindful approach to food, doing mini-meditations to check in with himself about his level of hunger and whether there were other reasons— stress, boredom, emotions—that were driving him to eat. He also learned to savor every aspect of the food he does eat, taking time to appreciate its appearance, smell, flavor, and texture. Instead of inhaling a sandwich in five bites, it now takes him twelve bites just to get through a piece of toast. This new approach, along with eating regular meals of home-cooked food and increasing his level of physical activity, has allowed him to drop sixty pounds. Tom's now lighter than he's ever been as an adult, more in touch with the motivations that drive his behavior, and, he would tell you, a lot happier, too.

Menu, Menu on the Wall

If knowledge equals power, and if nutrition labels are how consumers know what they're buying when shopping for groceries, how can they know what they're ordering when dining out—especially when it comes to calories? Yale University's Rudd Center for Food Policy & Obesity found that 80 percent of people wanted to know the nutritional content of the food they ordered when eating out.

In December 2006, the New York City Board of Health voted unanimously to require restaurants to offer just that with its proposal to make calorie information available on menus and menu boards. And the restaurant industry had a collective panic attack.

Many restaurants tried to avoid the requirement, by, for example, missing the deadline for turning in their sample menu boards. Dunkin' Donuts submitted a menu board designed to "prove" that calorie information couldn't fit. Some took it even further.

McDonald's, Burger King, Wendy's, and many others refused outright to comply with the law while the New York State Restaurant Association sued the city in Federal Court. Its claim? The menu labeling regulations violated restaurants' First Amendment free speech rights.

At the time, Margo Wootan, director of nutrition policy at the Center for Science in the Public Interest said, "It's shameful that the restaurant industry is working so hard to keep their customers in the dark. You've got to wonder what they are trying to hide."

In 2008, New York City prevailed. A proposal for menu labeling was enforced, and cities and states across the country began writing their own regulations. The saga reached a happy conclusion in 2010, when the federal health-care reform bill included a requirement that chains with more than twenty locations nationwide must implement menu labeling.

HEALTHY SUCCESS?

Subway was the first large chain to comply with the menu labeling laws. Did it hurt their sales? It's hard to know. By the end of 2010, Subway had surpassed McDonald's to become the world's largest restaurant chain—but it wasn't because menu labeling highlighted their lower-calorie options. When the New York City Department of Health conducted its initial studies of menu labeling in 2008, it found that Subway had undermined its customers' best calorie-counting intentions with a single step: It introduced the $5 Footlong sandwich.

While ordering a Footlong Veggie Delite without cheese, bacon, or sauce wouldn't be too bad, coming in at 440 calories, if you went instead for a Footlong Meatball Marinara with cheese and pepperoni on a 9-Grain Honey Oat bun, you'd be picking up 1,320 calories for your five-dollar deal. In the world of marketing, value trumps health any day, especially during a recession.

Menu (Mis)Labeling

The restaurant industry may have lost the battle against camouflaging unhealthy food, but they aren't done fighting the war. While they might be forced to display nutritional information, that's not the whole story.

The Energy Metabolism Laboratory of the USDA Human Nutrition Research Center at Tufts University tested 269 items from forty-two different restaurants and found sizable discrepancies in almost 20 percent of the calorie listings. And shockingly, most of the differences were from the low-calorie items. Restaurants underreported the calorie content of their healthiest entrees by an average of 100 calories, a significant difference to anyone trying to manage their weight.

The Blame Game

When asked about the role of restaurants in contributing to the obesity problem, Steven Anderson, president of the National Restaurant Association, stated, "Just because we have electricity doesn't mean you have to electrocute yourself."*

Corporate strategy often seeks to place responsibility on the people who consume products instead of on the parties who make and market them. Because the people who eat at restaurants are the customers whose health may be harmed, it seems like an ironic twist on biting the hand that feeds you.

10

Big Food Companies vs Us

No matter where you eat—in a fast-food restaurant, full-service restaurant, coffee shop, or at home—the majority of food you are consuming originates from the same sources: a handful of large global food companies.

The food industry consists in large part of massive agribusiness companies with staggering annual revenues, including Cargill ($120 billion) and Archer Daniels Midland ($81 billion); food manufacturers like Nestlé ($105 billion), Kraft ($49 billion), and PepsiCo ($60 billion); and restaurant companies like McDonald's ($24 billion) and Yum! Brands ($11 billion), which owns KFC, Pizza Hut, and Taco Bell. This industry is represented by lobbyists, lawyers, and trade organizations that in turn may represent a certain type of food (e.g., Snack Food Association, American Beverage Association), a segment of the industry (e.g., National Restaurant Association, Grocery Manufacturers of America), or even a single ingredient (e.g., Sugar Association, Corn Refiners Association).

Processed Profits

Success in food manufacturing, as in most businesses, is measured in profits. While many multinational food companies like Unilever and Kraft sell both healthy and unhealthy products, profit margins are usually much higher on processed foods. For example, healthy fresh fruits and vegetables are expensive to shepherd from seed to store, have a small window of peak color and taste, and go bad if not sold quickly enough, which wastes food and money. Food manufacturers would rather rely on commodity products, which can be processed into shelf-stable food products that we, as consumers, like.

But, in and of themselves, the artificial colors and flavoring in the processed foods we eat and the abundance of salt aren't making us fat. So why do we bring up their ingredients at all?

Without additives, instant chocolate pudding would have a greenish color and taste nothing like chocolate. Additives are also part of a marketing technique to make processed foods seem healthier and more attractive than they actually are. No child has ever harvested an actual berry from a bowl of Cap'n Crunch's Crunch Berries, but the cereal's bright colors and sweet scent mimic the signs of ripeness in nature enough to tempt both child and parent, at least subconsciously.

A DEFINING PROCESS

There are lots of definitions of "processed food"—for example, some might call baby carrots processed, since they have been cut and put into a bag. For our purposes, the processed foods we're referring to are the foods built from raw commodities (and from the meat raised on those same commodities), which food companies are able to break down and reconstruct into a wide variety of products. Think hot dogs, soda, cheese puffs, toaster pastries, corn chips, snack cakes, juice drinks, and whatever you'll find in the nearest vending machine.

The important thing to remember is that, in general, processed foods are much more likely to be loaded with the extra sugars and fats that are contributing to our obesity problem. If you limit or avoid processed foods, you'll probably be lowering your intake of the additional sugar and fat calories none of us need. Whole, healthy foods are usually better for you, and eating appropriate portions of those foods—fruits, vegetables, lean proteins, fat-free and low-fat dairy, and whole grains—will fill you up and deliver the fiber, vitamins, and other nutrients that your body needs, without the stuff you're better off without.

JUNK FOOD PAYS

Profit Margin for Fresh Produce = 10 percent
Profit Margin for Soft Drinks = 90 percent

Why is this a problem for you? While artificial ingredients themselves don't lead to weight gain, overconsumption does. Technological advances in food processing and packaging along with inexpensive artificial ingredients can increase food companies' opportunities to produce food in less expensive ways. In some ways, this is a good thing, especially for people who stretch every dollar to feed their families. But often we end up eating more and more of these products, which are loaded with the salt, sugar, and fat that we crave, and that overconsumption contributes to weight gain.

A good example is high-fructose corn syrup, commonly abbreviated HFCS. Yes, yes, you've heard way too much about it. We're not going to debate its health properties again—if it's really worse for you than sugar or if it's just about the same. There are plenty of scientific articles that cover those issues and more in great detail. What we want you to understand is why HFCS is such an appealing product to the food industry.

When the process of turning corn into a sweetener was patented in the late 1970s, food companies immediately began taking advantage of this new ingredient. Having a subsidized commodity crop like corn as the basis for a sweetener made HFCS much less expensive than sugar to produce and use.

Coca-Cola and PepsiCo took advantage of this opportunity to reduce their manufacturing expenses. The soda giants decided to use only HFCS to sweeten their drinks and other products in the early 1980s, saving 20 percent on their sweetener costs—literally billions of dollars (although research tells us that it made very little difference in price to the consumer).

But the switch from sugar to HFCS certainly didn't drive away many thirsty customers. Studies show that Americans now consume nearly three times as many calories from soft drinks as they did in the late 1970s. Today, almost a quarter of teens drink three or more sodas per day—the calorie equivalent of an entire extra meal.

Little Changes = **Big Results**

It's easy to get caught up in the intricacies of ingredient lists, wondering how much of any one component is in there, or what's behind those natural and artificial flavorings. One option for keeping it simple is to follow the advice of author Michael Pollan: Don't eat any processed food with more than five ingredients or that contains any ingredient whose name you can't pronounce!

Label Logic

Recently, food companies have responded to consumer demand for more choices of healthier products that offer lots of nutrients and fewer calories. This is a good thing. However, sometimes it is done in ways that are very confusing. Alleged "healthfulness" can often be used as a selling point for certain products that might not be as healthy as we think.

For example, when consumers learned how important whole grains were to a healthy diet, food manufacturers responded with more whole-grain products. However, some manufacturers and their advertising agencies began labeling many foods, from hot dog buns to spaghetti, as "multigrain" or "made with whole grain." Unfortunately, multigrain or "made with whole grain" does not necessarily mean 100 percent whole grain! "Multi" means more than one. Wheat, oats, and barley all start out as whole grains, but if they're refined, they lose much of the fiber that makes them healthy in the first place.

Misleading serving sizes also deter our best healthy intentions. An individual bag of potato chips may be listed as one serving; another similarly sized bag might read one and a half servings. If you don't check carefully, you could be eating 50 percent more than you planned.

And good luck finding a vending machine stocked with anything smaller than a twenty-ounce bottle of Coke. That's two and a half servings of soda, and not many of us stop even halfway through the bottle.

What is the problem with serving sizes being so variable? Well, a smaller serving size listed on a label can make a product appear to be healthier than it is. Nutrition information is listed per serving size, and the smaller the serving size, the smaller the calorie and fat counts will be. Not many of us stop to do these calculations of the total contents.

Fat-Free . . . For ¼ of a Second

The funniest serving-size example we know of? The makers of Pam cooking spray state on the can that a single serving size is a "¼ second spray." (Remember to count to ¼ second the next time you spray!)

But the manufacturers of Pam aren't trying to be funny. Instead, they're taking advantage of what amounts to a "fat-free" loophole in food labeling regulations. As long as there is half a gram or less of fat (or trans fat) *per serving*, manufacturers can label a serving as having 0 grams of fat! A can of olive oil spray, even when it contains 100 percent olive oil (which certainly has fat) can take advantage of this labeling loophole if the listed serving size is small enough. Coffee creamers that claim to have zero fat per serving may actually contain 40 percent fat, but if the serving size is listed as a teaspoon (which has less than 0.5 grams of fat)—an unrealistic serving size for many—it's perfectly okay to claim zero fat. If one teaspoon has 0.4 gram of fat and you use a tablespoon, that's 1.2 grams of fat—when you thought you were getting none.

Little Changes = **Big Results**

Want some of the healthiest foods of all? Buy the stuff that doesn't even have a nutrition label: apples, broccoli, spinach, bananas. . . .

Big Food = Big Tobacco?

Some experts believe there are a lot of similarities between Big Tobacco and what some now call major food manufacturers: Big Food. As Kelly Brownell of the Rudd Center for Food Policy & Obesity puts it:

> When the tobacco industry said smoking doesn't cause lung cancer, nicotine's not addictive, there's nothing, nothing bad about second-hand smoke, the government said, okay, well, we're not going to do anything because you're going to try to clean up your own act. And you could count the number of unnecessary deaths from all that stalling in the millions.

But Brownell cautions us to proceed carefully down this path: "Are we going to make that same mistake here with the food industry? Are we going to let them say they're doing good things when they're really not? And are we going to, as a country, just sit idly by while there's all kinds of unnecessary death and disability produced by diseases that could be prevented?"

As the comparisons between Big Tobacco and Big Food gain more ground, food manufacturers are recognizing that producing healthier products may help them bolster their reputations (while at the same time increasing profits as consumer demand for them grows).

What is important to know for your health and waistline is that just because a product has the aura of health food or is sold in your local Whole Foods doesn't mean it's low in calories, lacking in added sugars, fat, and salt, or that its redeeming nutritional qualities outweigh its bad ones. It doesn't matter where you buy it, whether its box is made from recycled cardboard, or what health claims it makes—processed food products are generally calorie-dense, nutrient-poor, and probably not the best choice. Buyer beware.

Food for Thought

It may not be fair to say that the food industry is trying to make us obese—but it is fair to say that the food industry's pursuit of profits is encouraging us to buy and consume more of their products—the over-consumption of which leads to the weight gain that threatens our personal health and the health of our nation.

You can become an educated consumer, which will help you, your family, and perhaps even the food companies themselves. While your personal knowledge will lead you to make healthier choices, demanding and encouraging the food industry to produce healthier products could lead to changes in the kinds of products that the food companies offer you and your fellow Americans. The food industry is resourceful, productive, and wants to be responsive to consumers. If we all demand better food, they will sell it to us!

11

Supermarkets vs Us

The average American spends more than 2,700 minutes a year grocery shopping. Retail supermarkets measure success not only in terms of overall sales—$464 billion in 2005—but also on a profit-per-square-foot basis. As an industry, supermarkets have a very low profit margin, and so they want to capitalize on every inch of their retail space. The majority of their product real estate, especially the prime locations like the ends of the aisles and front-of-store displays, are reserved for the products with the highest profit margins. The apple of a store's eye isn't usually fresh produce; too often, it's processed food.

Supermarkets make our lives easier by stocking a wide variety of foods, which allows us to do all our shopping in one place. They also often make it harder for us to make healthy choices about what to eat. In many respects, the modern supermarket is similar to a watering hole on the savanna, drawing hungry customers from miles around. Through their skilled use of marketing techniques, supermarkets purposefully engage many of our innate drives in order to make us buy more and buy certain products.

Designed to Sell

Many shoppers enter a supermarket to pick up a few items, such as ingredients for a salad to accompany the evening's meal; however, today's supermarkets are carefully designed so that you'll almost always leave with more than you came for. Paul Roberts, the author of *The End of Food*, explains, "The typical grocery store can make a sixth, maybe even a fifth of its profits from its produce section. But just as importantly, produce is a big magnet; it draws traffic. If you have a good produce section you'll bring people in and they'll buy more products, perhaps with even higher profit margins."

The average grocery store is 50,000 square feet, with large chain stores averaging more than 150,000. Fresh food is usually found along the perimeter of the store, leaving the bulk of the floor open to boxes, cans, and packaged, processed foods.

The idea is that, once you get past the produce, you'll be greeted by endless aisles in the center of the store filled with boxes of crackers, bags of chips, and cans of everything imaginable. Dr. Deborah Cohen, a senior scientist at the RAND Corporation, opens our eyes to an alarming statistic: "Almost 60 percent of all purchases in a supermarket are unplanned." There are several tricks of the retail trade that are used to lead consumers into making decisions without much thought. A primary example of this is "pseudovariety," or offering seemingly endless varieties of a certain product or brand. According to Dr. Cohen, "Doubling shelf space devoted to a particular item in a supermarket increases purchases by about 40 percent. So, when you go to a market, you look and see there's a whole aisle for sugar-sweetened beverages. There's a whole aisle for chips and salty snacks. And the reason that entire aisle exists is because it does increase what we buy." While you may not pick up a pack of the Oreo DoubleStuf Cakesters when browsing the cookie aisle, when you see the Oreo Peanut Butter Fudge Cremes a little farther down the shelf, you might just say, "That one's for me!"

Another way supermarkets encourage the purchase of a product is through positioning, by placing products where visibility will be increased, such as with end-of-aisle displays. Dr. Brian Wansink, director of the Cornell University Food and Brand Lab, explains: "It doesn't matter what it is, and it doesn't matter if it's on sale, but something on an end-of-aisle display can make you up to 30 percent more likely to buy it than if it's in the interior." Eye-tracking studies reveal that two-thirds of the attention we pay to end-of-aisle displays are because of the way they are designed. The edges, width, brands, colors, and way the displays are put together are among the factors that are meticulously arranged for maximum appeal.

Because of that, retailers drive a hard bargain for that space. They charge "slotting fees" to food manufacturers for the best spots in the store, and the ends of the aisles are among the most sought after. Guess who can afford those? Large food companies. And what do they want to sell? Their highest-margin foods: usually the sugary, processed kind. A smaller, independent company might come up with a healthier product, but unless the company can pay the price for the prime retail space in the store, consumers are unlikely to notice it. (Though if enough customers ask for a certain type of food, like locally grown vegetables or whole-grain breads from a local bakery, supermarkets might decide that those foods can also drive profits and stock them in a prominent position.)

Understanding that some shoppers will successfully navigate past that initial shiny end-of-aisle display, retailers are certain to stock the same food in multiple locations throughout the store. Deborah Cohen explains the reason for this: "If you miss it on the first aisle, it shows up again on the second or the third aisle to keep reminding you that this is something you needed to pick up. A lot of times people will automatically pick things up. They saw it before, now they see it again, and it's a cue that that was something they needed to put in their cart."

Little Changes = **Big Results**

To find the freshest food in the grocery store, focus on the perimeter, an idea nutritionist and food policy expert Marion Nestle has promoted for years.

But that's not just because most shoppers are likely to traverse the aisles of junk in order to make their way back to the milk. The fresh stuff is also placed around the edges of the store because that's what's restocked most frequently and the food delivery trucks have easier access to the perimeter.

While walking around the supermarket, you'll often be greeted by a friendly salesperson offering free food samples. This can be a welcome break for the hungry shopper, but what you may not realize is that this marketing triggers a sense of reciprocity. "If someone gives you something, you want to do something back for them," according to Dr. Cohen. "You just automatically want to reciprocate. And so that's really what happens when people give you a free sample. They give you something so you say to yourself, 'Oh, well, I'll just go ahead and buy the product in exchange.'"

Cross-merchandising, or pairing complementary foods, is another strategy supermarkets employ as a way of fetching profit. It isn't uncommon to see salad dressing in the produce case, peanut butter in the bread aisle, salsa alongside the chips, and chocolate sauce below the strawberries. For a consumer who was already planning to buy those items together, that might make it more convenient, but for those who only had strawberries on their list, the chocolate dipping sauce on the shelf below might just be too great a temptation. These are only a few examples of the many pairings that increase impulse purchase opportunities.

Playing to All Your Senses

It's not just what you see in the supermarket that can influence your purchase decisions; what you hear and feel also figure in. Studies in the 1970s and '80s found that when the music in a store was faster, people walked faster and bought less, but when the store played slower music, people took more time and sales increased nearly 20 percent. Stores also deliberately lower the thermostat to make you chilly and subliminally encourage you to "hoard" more food.

Perhaps the most important sense that supermarkets appeal to is our sense of value. Signs that offer multiple unit prices, like "5 for $5" or "Limit 12" often successfully tempt us into buying more. Dr. Wansink believes these cues influence even the most conscious shopper and will increase purchases, whether or not the product is truly on sale. Prior to entering the store, you may not have had soup on your radar at all, but after spotting it on sale, with a quantity limit, the perception that there's a time-sensitive bargain to take advantage of may convince you to stock up.

Check Your List Twice

Some customers think they are protected against these land mines because they go to the supermarket armed with a shopping list. According to Wansink, "The myth with lists is that you're going to be immune to impulse purchasing." That is not necessarily true because, as he says, "People who shop with lists are also the people who tend to reserve a big time in their day or week to go shopping. It's an event for them. So, as a result, they spend longer in the store. The longer you spend in the store, the more you buy."

Finally, there is one area of the supermarket everybody must pass through: the checkout aisles, or as Paul Roberts likes to call them, "canyons." Roberts says, "When you're walking through the canyons, you're going to be hemmed in on both sides by high-margin, impulse products." As in all other areas of the supermarket, positioning is key here, too. In many checkout lanes, mints and gum are placed closer to the top so they are directly in an adult's line of sight, while chocolates and candies are closer to the floor, making them easy for small children to grab and plead for. (Some stores have recently added non-candy checkout aisles to help parents with young children.)

Little Changes = Big Results

Supermarkets respond to the demands of their customers. So it's up to you to speak with your local supermarket's manager if they're not stocking the high-quality, healthy food you want to buy. That's how those new non-candy checkout aisles were born. Demand healthy, buy healthy, eat healthy!

The Opposite Problem

A large number of Americans don't have the option to shop at supermarkets, because they don't live anywhere near one. Experts believe that many low-income urban and rural areas have a higher percentage of obese residents in part because they live in "food deserts." These food deserts don't completely lack food, but they are generally devoid of supermarkets with fresh produce and other healthy options. Some areas are overpopulated with convenience stores and fast-food restaurants. The abundance of cheap, greasy, fatty foods often found in low-income neighborhoods has caused some to dub them "food swamps."

No matter what you call them, the areas with fewer grocery stores have a disproportionate number of public health problems. Accordingly, people from the community level up through the federal government have taken on eliminating food deserts as their cause. The Obama administration's new national Healthy Food Financing Initiative, based on a successful program piloted in Pennsylvania, provides incentives to supermarket owners to increase access to healthy, affordable foods in communities that currently lack them.

But supermarkets are a mixed bag of groceries. While they are a wonderful, essential part of all healthy communities, providing access to many things we need to maintain a healthy weight and eat our fruits and veggies, they also contain many unhealthy foods.

FRESH TO THE MASSES

In January 2011, Walmart, the nation's largest food retailer, announced a five-year plan to make thousands of its packaged, store-brand foods healthier and to lower prices on fruits and vegetables. According to Andrea Thomas, a senior vice president for sustainability at Walmart, "If we are successful in our efforts to lower prices, we believe we can save Americans who shop at Walmart approximately $1 billion per year on fresh fruit and vegetables."* Walmart came to the decision when it joined Let's Move!, the White House and First Lady Michelle Obama's campaign to end childhood obesity. Among its promises, Walmart is pledging to cut sodium by 25 percent, reduce added sugars by 10 percent, and eliminate all industrially added trans fats from its store brand, Great Value, by 2015. Walmart hopes its decision will help persuade major food suppliers to follow suit and help bring down the price of healthy food.

- 12 -

Marketing vs Us

The competition among food companies to be the market leader in America is fierce. Brands are forced to use every technique imaginable to maintain or advance their position. The major casualty in these battles among corporations? Our growing waistlines. In the forty-year war between Coke and Pepsi, corporate discussions have probably not been about the cuteness of the polar bear mascot or the sexiness of the new skinny can, but rather about the effectiveness of the marketing tools each company employs and whether they've allowed one to continue its reign or the other to unseat the undisputed king of soft drinks.

Increasingly, just a few large, global companies dominate our food world, and the stakes of dropping into second place can mean billions to them. So what's a billion here, a billion there, spent on marketing, if that's what it takes to increase profits?

Phil Marineau, former president of PepsiCo North America and the Quaker Oats Company, puts his own spin on an old advertising saw, attributed to everyone from Henry Ford to David Ogilvy, to describe how marketers throw everything at the wall and see what sticks when trying to build awareness of their product and drive sales: "I know at least half of my advertising works, I just don't know which half."

The food industry spends $30 billion every year on advertising—almost half of that exclusively on ads for snack foods, candy, and soda. And the advertising is working, especially on our kids.

Marketing vs Our Kids

A study conducted by the Rudd Center for Food Policy & Obesity at Yale University found that, while adults ate more following exposure to snack food advertising, children ate *a lot* more: 45 percent more. A recent Institute of Medicine report shows that, for children, there is strong evidence that marketing works to establish food preferences, increase requests for purchases, and drive up at least short-term consumption.

Research shows that children younger than age seven or eight do not have the cognitive abilities to understand that advertising is trying to sell a product and often have a hard time distinguishing it from regular programming. Children are trusting, easily persuaded, and incapable of resisting the sophisticated enticements of junk food consumption.

And they see a lot of enticements. Every day, our children see an average of fifteen TV commercials for food products—that's 5,500 ads for food commercials a year. And 98 percent of those are for foods high in fat, sugar, and salt. The commercials don't just hype how good the food tastes; they create lifelong associations of fun, good times, and being cool with the salty, fatty, sugary, colorful, appealing food that is usually unhealthy. As Kelly Brownell, the director of the Rudd Center, who has studied food marketing for years, describes it, "Food marketers are powerful, predatory, and pernicious in how they go after our kids." His colleague Marlene Schwartz adds, "If parents are going to succeed in managing the health of their children, they have to stop being undermined at every turn by food manufacturers."

RIGHT ON TARGET

In an attempt to influence and attract the greatest number of potential customers, the food industry, like many other industries, engages in what is known as "targeted marketing": creating custom advertising tailored to a certain demographic. Pepsi's "We Inspire" campaign is targeted at African American women, featuring celebrity spokespeople like Queen Latifah and Taraji P. Henson. Dr Pepper's "Vida23" campaign is aimed at bilingual Latino teens and young adults.

Billboards and other outdoor ads are also tailored to the neighborhoods in which they appear—and not every community has the same number of them. A team of researchers at UCLA and the University of Pennsylvania found that predominantly African American zip codes have the highest density of ads for high-calorie, unhealthy food; Latino neighborhoods have slightly fewer; and white areas have the least. When you consider that people in the neighborhoods with the most ads for unhealthy foods may also have the hardest time obtaining healthy food and are often mired in a food swamp filled with fast-food restaurants and convenience stores, it's no surprise that researchers suspect that targeted marketing contributes to the higher rates of obesity that these communities face.

Think Outside the Talking Box

The food industry doesn't limit its marketing to television alone. As our eyes drift away from billboards and subway ads, and we skip right through commercials on our DVRs, a growing share of every marketing budget is devoted to the digital domain and to alternative, often subtle ways of shaping our subconscious desires and consumer behavior. Mark Zuckerberg is not a billionaire because he helped you reconnect with your best friend from kindergarten, and Sergey Brin and Larry Page, co-founders of Google, didn't make their fortunes helping you research term papers. Every time you tweet about a Snickers Super Bowl commercial or join the more than 2 million other fans of Doritos on Facebook, you're doing marketers' work for them.

Along with the traditional fantasy-filled commercials and glossy magazine inserts, snack companies have upped their game, holding contests for aspiring musicians and filmmakers, sponsoring major charity events and concerts, and backing Olympic athletes. Pepsi has made a name for itself online by letting people vote for which local nonprofits should receive grants from its Refresh campaign. That's great for community organizations all over the country, but how good is it for our health? While it may feel warm and fuzzy to promote such a contest and raise money for a cause you care about, by participating in this campaign you're in effect providing free advertising for Pepsi.

Once again, all this marketing is especially effective at reaching our kids. In an effort to attract young consumers in less obvious ways, food manufacturers have turned to the digital marketplace to push their brands. Snack food and soda companies increasingly host online contests, promotions, and sponsorships in child-friendly areas of the web to speak to kids where their parents are less likely to be listening. The industry has even taken children's height into consideration, encouraging supermarkets to place the brightly colored boxes that kids find irresistible low to the ground in the cereal aisle, right at a kid's eye level. Pester power: Activated!

Even more subtle and pervasive advertising can be found right in your child's school. Soda companies offer free athletic equipment to physical education programs, along with large scoreboards in school gyms, all plastered with Coke or Pepsi logos. Cash-strapped elementary schools accept free reading material and educational posters from food companies like Chuck E. Cheese's, all of which are adorned with the brand's mascot. Other companies create extensive programs ostensibly aimed at promoting reading. The problem? The "reward" for students who meet their monthly reading goal in Pizza Hut's BOOK IT! program is a coupon for a free (590-calorie) personal pan pizza. McDonald's offers schools a percentage of an evening's sales profits from "McTeacher's Night," where teachers don McDonald's uniforms and sell burgers, fries, and soda to their students and their families at their local franchise.

Little Changes = **Big Results**

There's no question that the inactivity that results from children watching too much television should concern any parent. Increasingly, though, research is showing that the biggest problem with too much tube time isn't that it's turning our kids into couch potatoes, but that it's shaping the foods they crave, what they're willing to eat, and what they beg you to buy them.

Dr. Elsie Taveras, a Harvard pediatrician who studies this problem, says, "Evidence is showing that television viewing is related to weight gain and obesity because kids are exposed to toxic advertising." The American Academy of Pediatrics now recommends zero screen time for children younger than two, and no more than one to two hours a day of quality (ad-free) programming for older kids.

If you cut back TV viewing to these levels, you greatly reduce the chances of a temper tantrum when you make a healthy choice in the cereal aisle or a meltdown as you drive past the Golden Arches.

An Uphill Battle

To help put the scope of food marketing in perspective, it's interesting to note that the Robert Wood Johnson Foundation, the nation's largest public health philanthropy, made history's largest commitment to reverse child obesity trends in 2007, when it pledged $100 million per year for five years. The food industry spends more than that marketing junk food to our children *every month*.

The USDA spent $220 million in 2004 on nutrition education. That's merely 2 percent of what the food industry spent to market its products to our kids that same year.

Researchers have calculated that a ban on fast-food advertising during children's television programming could reduce the number of overweight children by 18 percent. In 2009, Congress tasked the Federal Trade Commission (FTC), the Food and Drug Administration (FDA), the USDA, and the CDC with developing a set of *voluntary* steps the food industry could take to limit the marketing of unhealthy food to children. Industry objected, and in 2011 after soliciting testimony from policy experts and industry spokespeople, Congress landed on the side of industry and sent the guidelines back to the drawing board. In that congressional hearing to review the draft standards, Representative Marsha Blackburn (R-TN) said, "The government should stop pretending after all these decades that it has the answer because it does not."

Yet another failed attempt to help parents do the right thing for their children.

DEW THE MATH

In 2006, the American Beverage Association said its members were no longer advertising high-sugar drinks during children's television programs. An investigation by the Rudd Center for Food Policy & Obesity at Yale discovered that companies were narrowly defining both the drinks that were banned and the programs that were deemed off-limits, advertising more during other programs children watch. From 2008 to 2010, the number of advertisements for non-diet soda viewed by children and teens across all programming actually doubled.

13

The Fashion and Beauty Industries vs Us

If you're doing this to look good, if your motivation is to fit into a skinnier pair of jeans, we've got bad news for you: Chances are, you are going to be among the 95 to 98 percent of people who regain the weight they lose (and more) after dieting. Successfully maintaining a significant weight loss requires a serious attitude adjustment and a lifelong commitment to changing the way you live—not the way you look.

The fashion and beauty industries aren't interested in your health. Like any other industry, they're in business to make a profit, and they do that by selling clothes, beauty products, and magazines. If you're going to succeed at transforming your life and your health, you have no choice but to reconcile your relationship with fitting rooms, mirrors, and movie stars.

The majority of Americans are overweight or obese because we live in a world that is poorly suited to the biology we inherited. We must recognize and account for that, but our ultimate goal should be one thing: a healthy body.

Like our hair, skin, and facial features, healthy bodies come in many varieties. Our goal as a nation should be to embrace the bodies we were born with. There's no such thing as a perfect body, but there is such a thing as a healthy one.

Not all healthy women will fit into size 4 jeans. Not all healthy men will be able to bench press their weight. But a healthy body will give you the greatest chance of being able to enjoy your life, and the lives of your kids, your grandkids, and even your great-grandkids.

A Perfect Fit?

Elana, the video editor profiled in chapter 6 who lost more than a hundred pounds, sums up the feelings of many overweight and obese women when she describes how traumatic an experience shopping for clothes can be: "First of all, I shopped as little as possible. When I did go, every time I got in the dressing room, I literally would be drowning in tears."

Each pair of pants that's too tight to pull all the way up and each dress that reveals all your bulges is another ding to your self-esteem. But you don't have to approach it that way. Catalog all the reasons you love yourself: your smarts, your ambition, your good nature, your loyalty, your dreams and aspirations. At a minimum, clothes are a tool for staying warm, and while they do play into our natural desire to appear attractive, you don't have to let them take control of your life. If the pants don't fit, just try on another pair.

Your looks shouldn't be first on your list of reasons why you want to lose weight. Your health, longevity, and happiness clearly matter much more. But we're not denying that looks play a role, too, and can enhance happiness, so we're not suggesting you strike them off your list entirely. As you put in all the hard work required to lose weight and buckle down for the long term to keep it off, remember that your healthy new outlook can bring you a whole new look, as well.

Now that she's back down to a healthy weight, Elana says, "The difference is now, everything I bring into the dressing room fits me, looks beautiful, every single thing. The tears still come, but now out of gratitude."

What They Know That You Don't

Fashion 101 isn't a requirement in American education, but, if it were, it might help explain some of what goes on behind the velvet ropes and runway curtains, and why.

Karl Lagerfeld, head designer and creative director at Chanel, once famously said that fashion was all to do "with dreams and illusions." This is an industry where excess and the unattainable are embraced and celebrated.

When you flip through a glossy magazine and see a stylish Angelina Jolie floating down a river in Cambodia, you may know you'll never look like her, or even visit a country in Southeast Asia, but perhaps you could be as chic. The business of fashion isn't just one of selling T-shirts and skirts; they are in the business of selling the intangible, an idea, a lifestyle, a goal. We all have a picture in our minds of our very best selves, and their job is to take that picture and edit it to include what they are offering.

If you could see deep into those pages to the inner workings of any major fashion magazine, you would know that, as important as it is to secure Mario Testino and Kate Moss for a shoot, the skilled Photoshop editor who painted that picture just so is perhaps even more crucial to the spread's success. These are the magicians who shave inches off thighs, enhance bust lines, tan skin, and smooth wrinkles in the blink of an eye. Fashion industry insiders know that the images we are looking at in magazines are nothing like what exists in real life.

Designers say they favor slender models to show off their clothes because the clothing hangs on them like it does on hangers. The average model has a two- to five-year career span, and it's likely that many of these rail-thin "hangers" rely on cigarettes, diet soda, and a generally unhealthy lifestyle to keep them looking as waifish as possible. If you head backstage at a fashion show you may see a catered spread, but in the industry it's widely understood that when food is present, it is there to be seen and not consumed. Keep in mind, this is the same industry that introduced the "heroin chic" look in the 1990s. This type of obsessive thinking is skewed and damaging both to the mind and body because, as is the case with anything so extreme, deprivation of this magnitude leads to serious issues with body image, self-esteem, and, in grave cases, eating disorders.

While it is perfectly fine to appreciate fashion and all the gorgeous textiles gracing the runways in Paris and Milan, it's smart to think of it more as fantasy or art than as something you should emulate or strive to attain in your own life.

Pants on Fire

Think you know your waist size because you know your pants or jeans size? Think again. While it makes sense that, for both women and men, a size 32 would mean a thirty-two-inch waist, it doesn't make for good sales when the average person's waist is bigger than that. Enter "vanity sizing," a legal trick clothing manufacturers employ to make customers feel better about themselves.

In reality, the actual waist measurements on pants all marked the same size can differ by as much as five inches.

How does this hurt us? By fooling us into believing we haven't gained weight because we still wear the same size 32 we always have, when in reality the clothes are keeping pace with our expanding waistlines.

The only sure way to know your waist size is to measure it yourself. The average for American women in 2011? Thirty-four and a half inches.

The oft-cited anecdote that Marilyn Monroe wore a size 10 has made many women feel better about their own (over)weight. But in the 1950s, a size 10 wasn't the same size 10 it is today. To keep pace with the growing American waistline, clothing manufacturers have simply shifted their measurements up while keeping the sizes down.

In the 1950s, a size 10 dress was made to fit a twenty-three-inch waist. Marilyn's measurements as recorded by her dressmaker were 36-23-37, with her waist sometimes expanding to twenty-four inches. Today a twenty-three-inch waist is a size 0 (and the average waist size of an eight-year-old girl).

Inner Beauty

We're not suggesting that you stop shopping. We all have to navigate the world of clothing stores, beauty counters, and newsstands. And we all want to look good and feel good about ourselves. But the way to get there is not by obsessing about our looks. Taking the lessons of this book to heart and applying them to your life is your best chance for achieving your goals. You'll feel better from the inside out, and everyone will tell you how good you look.

14

Desks, Cars, and Computers vs Us

Unless you're reading this while on the treadmill, you've probably just cut a few seconds off your life. Why? Because sitting, scientists have recently discovered, may be hazardous to your health.

Thanks to suburban sprawl, long commutes, and desk-bound jobs, most of us now spend most of our time away from home sitting. And when we are home, we have remotes to change the thousands of channels on our flat-screen TVs, microwaves to zap our frozen meals, and appliances to do our dirty work for us. People who study human behavior would call us sedentary. Dr. David Nathan, a Harvard diabetes expert, wonders if our legs are becoming vestigial limbs: "We won't need them after a while because nobody walks anymore." Technically, you are being sedentary any time you are expending less than 1.5 MET, or metabolic equivalent of tasks, a measure of how much energy an activity burns when compared to doing nothing at all. Working on a computer, driving, studying, or watching TV all fall under that category.

The average American adult is sedentary more than eight hours a day, about half the time we're awake. Kids spend 70 percent of their time in school being sedentary; add the six-plus hours a day of TV, computer use, and thumbs-only video gaming that they average, and you start to see the problem.

The Sitting Dead

It's not news to our bad backs and protruding posteriors that we sit a lot. What is startling is that the sedentary lifestyle may be killing us. And, apparently, not slowly.

In 2009, doctors at the Pennington Biomedical Research Center at Louisiana State University tried to determine in a study of seventeen thousand people whether there is any connection between how much time people spend sitting and their mortality rate. Even after accounting for age, smoking, and physical activity levels, they found that the most sedentary people were almost 50 percent more likely to die at a younger age than the least sedentary. Even worse: Exercising around those sedentary periods didn't make them any less harmful. If you work out at the gym for an hour before work and then sit for the next seven hours straight, you will likely share the same higher mortality rate as your coworkers who didn't hop on the elliptical this morning.

Why? It's more than just going a long time without moving. Sedentary behavior leads to sudden and startling physiological changes in your skeletal muscle and metabolism whether you're fat or lean. The American Heart Association warns that physical inactivity induces dramatic levels of insulin resistance and important changes to the health of our circulatory system. Monitoring healthy subjects after just five days of bed rest, the researchers found that their levels of triglycerides (a type of blood fat) had increased by 35 percent and insulin resistance by 50 percent.

Research in animals has shown that, after just six hours of sedentary behavior, a drastic decrease occurs in the activity of an enzyme that allows muscles to take fat out of the bloodstream.

Work or Workout?

On average, Americans spend 8.5 hours a day at work, and 4.5 hours a week doing extra work from home.

While the amount of time we spend at work hasn't changed too much over the years, the amount of physical energy we expend at work has—drastically. In the early 1960s, almost 50 percent of private sector jobs required at least moderate levels of activity. Today, less than 20 percent of jobs do.

Our Cars, Ourselves

The U.S. Census Bureau reports that Americans now spend more than one hundred hours a year commuting. That's 25 percent longer than the average vacation allowance. We're spending two and a half weeks per year driving to and from work. Sitting in traffic. And frequently eating to stay awake, fight boredom, fit in a meal between appointments, or divert our anger toward the driver who just cut us off.

Little Changes = **Big Results**

If you can get from home to work using public transportation instead of driving, try it. Not only can it be lighter on your wallet, it will be better for the planet—and it could also be an easy way to incorporate activity into your life. A recent nationwide study shows that 29 percent of transit users are active for thirty minutes or more each day, just by walking to and from public transit stops. Adults who use public transportation take 30 percent more steps and walk eight minutes more per day than those who drive.

Walking to and from the bus stop or subway station is a little change you can make to improve your health, start losing weight, or keep it off.

TV Time

Whether we love watching football, reality shows, or the latest groundbreaking series on HBO, television offers us more choices than it ever has before. Despite the allure of iPads and Kindles, we're not all throwing our TVs to the curb. American adults now watch an average of four hours of TV a day. And one study found that children ages 8 to 18 watched four and a half hours every day—and when researchers added up all their hours of media exposure (computers, music, video games, and movies) it amounted to more than ten hours. More time sitting. More opportunities to snack. More time watching ads for unhealthy food. In fact, one study found that children with a TV in their bedroom were 31 percent more likely to be overweight than children from a similar socioeconomic background without a TV in their bedroom.

Little Changes = **Big Results**

Don't eat in front of the TV. Just don't do it. We know it's hard, but set a rule for yourself and your family, and then stick to it. You're more distracted, more stimulated by tantalizing food commercials, and more likely to overeat because you're not paying attention to your food.

Don't Just Sit There!

To lower your risks of chronic diseases, boost your health, and lose weight, you don't have to quit your job and become a lumberjack. You don't need to ride your bike to work—though that's not a bad idea. You don't have to boycott March Madness or delete your Facebook account. Simply set an hourly alarm on your computer, watch, or phone to remind you to get up, stretch, and walk around for just five minutes. Researchers have found that taking small, frequent breaks can improve cholesterol levels, glucose tolerance, BMI, and waist circumference. They concluded it's the prolonged, uninterrupted sitting that's the most detrimental.

Other steps you can take to inject activity back into your life? Park your car ten or fifteen minutes from your office, walk the rest of the way, and then take the stairs. Or cook one more meal a week from scratch, because not only will the food you prepare be healthier, and probably tastier, but you burn calories just by moving around the kitchen, chopping, slicing, and dicing.

15

School Budgets vs Our Kids

If you are concerned about your child's weight and health, one important thing you can do is to eat lunch with him or her in the school cafeteria. And do it more than once. Chances are, it's not the school lunch you remember from your childhood. If you're not happy with what you see (or what you eat), you have to understand how we got here before you take action.

School Lunch 101

Obesity was the farthest thing from anyone's mind when the National School Lunch Act was passed in 1946. During the Great Depression, an abundance of underfed and hungry American schoolchildren had prompted the government to begin donating surplus commodity foods, like beef, milk, and other dairy products, to schools. After World War II, alarmed by the number of young people who had been rejected for military service because of malnourishment, legislators decided to institutionalize the school lunch program and placed it under the jurisdiction of the U.S. Department of Agriculture (USDA). In addition, they added cash reimbursements to the schools for each lunch served and directed the USDA to develop a meal pattern for the lunches based on scientific research.

Through the 1950s, '60s, and '70s, as the nation's economy expanded and income inequality grew, the need to feed America's hungriest and neediest children continued to be a priority.

In the 1980s, a conservative government slashed school meals funding by more than $1 billion. At the same time, communities across the country were cutting local taxes, which among other things, are one of the major sources for education funding in the nation. So, at the same time that school lunch funds had been cut, so were the funds that had previously supported other aspects of the school lunch program, like the wages of food service workers, their benefits, and equipment costs.

Although school administrators and school boards expected school food programs to stay in the black, they were not seen as part of the educational process, but rather as a service like custodial services and school buses. This put enormous pressure on school lunch programs and their managers to find ways to make ends meet while still feeding children. Many districts closed school kitchens or removed appliances other than microwaves and fryers and cut back on staff, relying on outside vendors or a bulk central kitchen to provide them with ready-to-serve food. Where once water fountains and cartons of milk were all they needed to offer kids, many school districts began selling exclusive "pouring rights" to beverage companies in exchange for vending machines stocked with only their branded products. At the same time, because pressure was increasing on the entire school budget, schools were often willing to make up for shortfalls by selling ad space on scoreboards and depending on outside companies' funding or their students' purchases of sugar-sweetened beverages to sponsor sports teams or other aspects of student life that had been taken for granted but were no longer affordable. Some schools even took food companies up on their offers of free branded textbooks for the classroom.

Then, fast-forward to 2007, when the USDA's most recent evaluation of the National School Lunch Program found that 94 percent of American schools failed to meet federal standards for healthy meals. How did we go from turkey, mashed potatoes, and carrots to Hot Pockets?

For the most part, lunches met and often exceeded the vitamin and mineral requirements but failed in the areas of fat, saturated fat, and sodium. When the Center for Science in the Public Interest (CSPI), a consumer advocacy group, evaluated the healthfulness of the nation's school food program around the same time, the average grade given was a D+.

Passing the Buck

Some politicians have argued recently that the health of our children is not the schools' problem.

In April 2011, in response to the USDA's call for better nutrition standards for school lunches, Congressman John Kline (R-MN), chairman of the House Education Committee, wrote that he did not believe the federal government should dictate what children eat: "That presupposes the only way you can address childhood obesity or get responsible behavior on the part of adults is to have a law from Washington, D.C. I fundamentally reject that notion."

While it's not the only way to address childhood obesity, it does make sense to look at where children are spending the majority of their time and consuming up to half their calories. For more than 55 million American kids, that place is school.

Kids spend more time at school than anywhere else outside their home. School breakfast and lunch programs may contribute to more than 50 percent of children's caloric intake on school days, and, when in class, kids sit, sit, and sit some more. Our children not only don't get regular gym class (only 4 percent of elementary schools have a daily physical education program), but many schools have also eliminated recess.

A Captive Audience

While adults can choose to enter a restaurant or not, and to hit the gym during a lunch break or not, children are required by law to go to school.

They aren't required to eat the school's food, but for 31 million of them, the free or reduced-price lunch program is the only way they can afford to eat lunch. For 20 million of those kids, school breakfast and lunch might be the only meals they eat in a day.

Ellen Carlson, whose son attends elementary school in Madison, Wisconsin, is a co-founder of Madison Families for Better Nutrition. As she sums it up:

> They are responsible for my child when he is there. And so they're responsible that they're giving him real food. If they're filling his body full of things, they should be filling his body full of real food.
>
> I know others have done it, and I expect that they will see the best interest of our kids and that they won't take the shortcuts. They'll find a way to get fresh food to our kids because that's their job.

So how are schools handling that job?

The Healthy Hunger-Free Kids Act

What Ellen Carlson hopes for when it comes to better school meals for her kids is now within reach due to a lot of dedicated work by people who care, but there have been a number of obstacles along the way. You may have heard that Congress recently declared pizza a "vegetable" in terms of school lunch, but the story is more complicated than you might think. In this case, it shows how the food industry can directly, and negatively, influence what our kids eat for lunch at school.

In December 2010, Congress passed the Healthy Hunger-Free Kids Act, which outlined the most substantial improvements to the school food program in a generation. The bill instructed the USDA to rewrite the regulations that govern the healthfulness of meals served to the 31 million American children who eat school lunches, based on recommendations from the Institute of Medicine. In response, the USDA proposed a slew of improvements to the program. Their primary recommendations were to change school lunches to include more fruits and vegetables (especially dark green and orange ones), fewer starchy vegetables (like potatoes), more whole grains, and less salt. For instance, under the previous guidelines, two tablespoons of tomato paste counts as one serving of vegetables in a school lunch. The USDA wanted to up that amount to a healthier ½ cup. However, while two tablespoons of tomato paste fits nicely on a slice of pizza, a half cup will not.

The frozen food companies that benefit substantially from the $11 billion school lunch budget were not happy with this turn of events, since it could hurt their bottom line. They spent upwards of $450,000 lobbying Congress against upping the tomato paste requirement, and Congress bowed. Our representatives decreed that the current amount of tomato paste—not technically the "pizza," with its bread, cheese, and pepperoni—would still count as a vegetable.

Looking back to December 2010, parents were probably pleased when Michelle Obama's efforts to pass the Healthy Hunger-Free Kids Act prevailed. But they, along with the First Lady, must have been less than thrilled that, in addition to the frozen food lobby succeeding at keeping pizza on kids' lunch trays by counting the two tablespoons of tomato paste as a vegetable serving, the potato lobby won a victory of its own when it, too, weakened the legislation. Potatoes count as a vegetable, even in the form of french fries, which is how they most frequently appear in the School Lunch Program. The USDA had recommended limiting starchy vegetables like potatoes to no more than two servings per week, but the potato lobby proved the power of the spud, and schools across the country can continue to serve up fries and tater tots every day (and many likely will, unless enough parents complain).

VEGETABLE SURPRISE

The debate about the types and amounts of products that count as a serving of vegetables in the school lunch program is nothing new. In 1981, at the request of President Reagan, Congress slashed the school lunch budget by $1 billion, and the USDA was instructed to find a way to reduce the cost of providing lunch. To save money, they tried to change the school lunch rules to, among other things, count ketchup as a vegetable (and relish, too), and reduce the amount of fruits, vegetables, and milk that schools needed to serve children. Thankfully, these proposed changes did not make it into the standards because of a major public outcry.

Despite some setbacks, the changes that remain for what's on the tray and the changes still to come to what other food can be sold in schools will go a long way toward improving what our kids eat. If the federal government sets standards, all states have to meet them—but there's nothing to say they can't exceed them, and at least twenty states already do.

And there's definitely nothing stopping your local school district, or even just your school, from dishing up fresh, delicious, locally grown meals full of lean protein, vegetables, whole grains, and ripe, juicy fruit or from banning the sale of junk food and selling only water and skim milk. All it takes is the desire to do so, a commitment to carrying it out, some ingenuity to figure out the finances, and advocacy to make it happen.

The USDA itself knows this can be done. To encourage schools that participate in the National School Lunch Program across the nation to up their game, it created the Healthier U.S. Schools Challenge, awarding bronze, silver, gold, and gold with distinction prizes to schools that created healthier school environments through the promotion of nutrition and physical activity. More than two thousand schools across the nation have already received recognition.

Little Changes = Big Results

Convince your school food service director to take up the Healthier U.S. Schools Challenge and get people in your community to support your school in this important effort. (The food service director may be willing, but the school administration, the school board, and the community also need to be behind the effort and understand its importance for it to succeed.) Go to hbo.com/theweightofthenation to find out more.

Hot Competition

Never heard of "competitive foods"? That's the official name for all food presented to schoolchildren outside of, or in competition with, the federally funded lunch program. There are two main categories of competitive foods: the alternative entrées like burgers and chicken fingers, often with fries, that tempt students away from the standard meal available as part of the National School Lunch Program; and the snacks, sodas, juice, and sports drinks that are available for purchase in and outside of the cafeteria. Many elementary schools have eliminated competitive foods entirely. However, middle and high school students still face the gauntlet of candy and soda vending machines lining their hallways, the racks of chips and cookies that flank the cash registers, and school stores that raise much-needed funds for clubs and teams by selling junk food. These foods generate extra profit for schools, provide great marketing for the food companies, and prove almost impossible for children and teens to resist. Would you have used the change in your pocket for carrot sticks instead of a Snickers when you were twelve? (How about now?)

Little Changes = Big Results

Do your kids use a school debit card to pay for lunch? If so, do you know what they are buying? Chances are, you'd be shocked by how many times a week little Ethan is swiping his way to an ice cream sandwich and a bag of chips.

How you manage this family financial matter is up to you, but if your child is busting his calorie budget on snacks at school, he's going to pay later.

USDA surveys tell us that in 2004 competitive foods were in 73 percent of our nation's elementary schools, 97 percent of the middle schools, and 100 percent of the high schools. And, on average, they add an extra 200 calories to a kid's daily consumption.

THE PROOF IS IN THE POUNDS

A program in Pennsylvania called the School Nutrition Policy Initiative targeted the weight problems of fourth through sixth graders in socioeconomically challenged areas. Their innovations were fairly simple: They removed all sugar-sweetened beverages and unhealthy snack foods from schools, set up a social marketing campaign to encourage the consumption of nutritious foods, and included parent outreach programs. In two years, the incidence of overweight among children who participated in the program was only 50% of the rate among children who weren't in the program. In less technical terms, this means that the program was effective at cutting the rate of new cases of overweight in half.

Let's Get Physical

The quality of school lunches isn't the only thing that has declined since you graduated from high school.

"Many of us remember growing up in school settings where we had to change into our gym uniforms three, four times, five times a week," says Dr. Elsie Taveras, a Harvard researcher and pediatrician at Children's Hospital in Boston. "There's been a pretty significant change in that."

And that may be an understatement. Despite the Physical Activity

Guidelines for Americans, which recommend children get a minimum of sixty minutes a day of moderate-to-vigorous physical activity, fewer than one in six schools across the country require PE at least three days a week for kids in all grades. Only a quarter of teenagers in public school are required to take any PE at all. And the numbers for daily PE are even worse—only 4 percent of elementary schools, 8 percent of middle schools, and 2 percent of high schools provide daily PE for their students. In fact, many schools have eliminated mandatory PE—and recess—altogether. In or out of school, less than one-third of all children get even twenty minutes of activity a day.

"When children are not burning as many calories, it makes it difficult for them to remain in energy balance," says Christina Economos, the nutrition researcher at Tufts University. "This lack of activity is also setting a pattern. If you're an inactive child, you're likely to grow up to be an inactive adult."

Little Changes = Big Results

Convince your child's teacher to set aside five to ten minutes during class time throughout the day for activity breaks. Go to hbo.com/theweightofthenation for some simple and fun activity suggestions.

PE Gets KO'd

Budget cuts to schools across the country left physical education programs feeling the same pressure as school cafeterias. Administrators found the success of their schools being judged solely on test scores, and began moving funding away from PE to focus on academic subjects like reading and math. CDC Director Dr. Thomas Frieden explains:

There's a tension. Principals will say, well, I can't increase the number of PE classes, because I've got to get the math and reading scores up. That's really misguided. If kids are getting physical activity on most or all days, they're going to learn better in class.

In fact, there are a number of studies showing that increased physical activity in schools actually helps kids learn and leads to better test scores. And to counter the concerns of principals who think there isn't enough time in the day to teach kids reading and math as well as have them run around the track, even short activity breaks during classes have been shown to improve academics and reduce behavior problems. As Dr. Frieden says, "If kids aren't bouncing up and down in gym, they're going to be bouncing off the walls in class."

GYM CLASS HERO

As with healthy school lunches, states and school districts drive the bus when it comes to standards for PE.

For nearly a decade, Susan Combs, the Texas state comptroller, has used her authority and years of legislative experience to try to make the Texas school environment healthier for the 4 million kids in her state.

"When children are in school," Combs says, "school administrators stand in the shoes of the parents. When the school itself does not promote or prompt physical activity, then that teaching moment for those children about a lifetime of fitness is absolutely lost."

In 2007, using her influence as comptroller, she took action, making millions of dollars in grants available to help Texas middle schools buy equipment for PE activities and create daily thirty-minute PE classes. Her big play has been a home run, both for children's health and for academics. Detailed data gathered from the thousands of children benefiting from these additional PE programs have shown improvements in fitness and academic performance.

PART IV

|||||||||||||||||||||||||||||||||

How to Lose Weight and Make It Last

We know we've rocked your world. We've just told you that so many of the things we love and take for granted may not be good for our health. You probably think we've asked you to question every time you order that piece of cheesecake, plant yourself on the couch for an entire Sunday of football, or share a jumbo tub of popcorn with your kids during the latest Hollywood blockbuster. You probably hate us by now and wish you had never bought this book. But here is where we assure you that we're not trying to sap all the joy out of your life—we're giving you the tools you need to live a healthier one.

We point out the sweet, fatty cheesecake, the lazy Sunday afternoon, and the salty popcorn because sometimes it helps to be reminded that we're biologically programmed to love those things. And we love them so much that we've made them part and parcel of our progress as a civilization.

Until recently, though, there were a few remote corners of the world not yet reached by modernity, where people still lived much the same way that our ancestors did for the majority of human history. Anthropologists who studied these groups in places like the South Pacific, the Amazon, and the far reaches of Siberia found a near-complete absence of heart disease, stroke, diabetes, and many other conditions, including obesity. Dr. Staffan Lindeberg of the University of Lund in Sweden, who has studied groups in Papua New Guinea for decades, observed the Western diet sweep across the island. As each tribe stopped hunting and started shopping—consuming for the first time a diet high in added sugars, fat, and salt—heart disease made its first appearance. Until recently, these communities had rarely seen someone die suddenly of a heart attack or stroke. Their language actually had no words to describe the experience. If a Papua New Guinean escaped infection, accident, and the perils of childbirth, it is believed that he or she would then live out the full natural lifetime of the human organism, remaining vital well into his or her nineties, even without the benefit of modern medicine.

The cautionary tale for all of us is that the arrival of the markets that transformed the diets of these people and the technology that enabled them to put down their hoe and spear can be viewed as a natural experiment showing the toll the Western diet and sedentary lifestyle are taking. The Papua New Guineans are no more able to turn down the cheesecake or turn off the TV than we are.

Huge numbers of us now have more food than we could have ever imagined, available at any hour, whether by ordering delivery online or pulling up to a drive-through window. This is the product of tremendous success on the part of our species. But that success has unintended consequences. And the unintended consequence we care most about here is that we are all at risk of living a shorter, sicker life.

The rest of this book is devoted to helping you have the best chance of living a longer, healthier, and, we hope, happier life.

By now, we're fairly certain you've gotten the message that the key to weight loss is to eat less and move more. It's very easy to say that, but for so many of us, it's incredibly hard to do. At this point, you understand why that is: There are strong forces at work inside our bodies and in the world around us that make it harder than it has to be.

But knowing what you're up against is the first step toward taking a stand. In the final four chapters, we build on the foundation we've given you so far to help you launch your own campaign against the things in your life and the systems in your body that are preventing you from achieving your optimal weight. If you're going to lose, you have to win that fight. And we believe you can do it.

In the not-too-distant future, when someone asks you how you lost all that weight, you can smile knowingly and say: I ate a little less and moved a little more. That's my secret.

16

What Not to Do—And What to Do About It

The IOM reports that even when people do lose weight by dieting, most of them regain two-thirds of what they lost within a year and all of it back within five. When an approach is so certain to fail, why try it at all?

We're going to say it here and now: It's time for America to stop dieting as we know it. No more cutting our caloric intake so low that we're practically starving ourselves, no more scrapping entire food groups in the service of some haphazard philosophy that promises to make us thin, no more blind hope that the latest fad approach will be the one that works. You'll never again read another diet column, watch another weight-loss infomercial at 2 A.M., take another diet pill, or spend thousands of dollars on a diet plan consisting predominantly of frozen meals endorsed by some TV star or athlete.

You have just bought your last diet book. You might be dismayed to find that you've gotten this far, and we haven't given you a diet either.

And we're not going to. That's because, for most of us, diets just don't work for the long term. And losing and regaining and losing and regaining is not a way that any of us should ever live again. Think of this instead as an anti-diet book.

If you make adjustments—often small ones—to what you consume and how much physical activity is in your life, you will slowly but surely start to see the number on the scale go down. And if you make those changes a part of your lifestyle, you may be able to beat the odds and say good-bye to your excess weight for the long term.

Myth #1: I Have to Lose It All

Many overweight and obese people think they have to lose all their extra weight to be healthy. According to what scientists have learned over the last thirty years, that's just not true. Researchers have found that a 7 to 10 percent weight loss is usually sufficient to significantly reduce your risk of developing diabetes, high blood pressure, and heart disease or to greatly improve those conditions if you already have them. If you need to lose more and manage to drop an even more admirable 20 or 30 percent of your weight, life just keeps getting better. Not only will you be far healthier, but you'll also likely have fewer aches and pains; move more easily, making exercise that much more fun and rewarding; and feel better about yourself and how you look. You may even feel like dancing.

If the notion that you had to get back down to what you weighed in high school in order to be healthy was so daunting that it held you back from even trying, fear no more. The greatest health benefits come from the first 10 percent of body weight you lose.

Myth #2: I'll Just Starve Myself for a Few Weeks

To lose that all-important 7 to 10 percent without throwing your body into all-out starvation-defense mode and having it sabotage all your efforts, you have to make peace with the fact that healthy, sustainable weight loss means about one to two pounds a week (except for the extremely obese, who may be able to lose at a faster rate, under a doctor's supervision). On the plus side, at that rate, it's much more likely that the pounds you're losing are actual fat and not just water weight!

Cut too many calories to try to shave off five pounds for the weekend, and your body will hit a brick wall as the caveman-era genetics that still control your biology will slow down your metabolism to ride out the perceived "famine." (If this sounds unfamiliar to you, you might want to go back and reread chapter 6, "Know Thy Body," for a quick refresher.)

Yes, that means it will take at least three months—and maybe longer—to lose about twenty pounds. But when thinking about a lifetime of better health, three months is nothing. If your sole motivation is to fit into the swimsuit, the wedding dress, or the tux, you may succeed at looking good on the beach or at your wedding, but the odds are two in three that by next summer you won't be so ready to flaunt it at the beach, and there's a 98 percent chance that by your fifth anniversary fitting into what you wore at your wedding will be a long-forgotten dream. Until you realize that your weight could be leading you to a shorter, sicker life, you're going to have a hard time mustering the patience you need to hold a slow and steady course. You didn't gain this weight overnight, and you cannot expect to lose it overnight, either, and lose it for good. The little changes you need to make to get the big results have to become a permanent part of your life.

A crash diet is simplistic. A lifestyle transformation is realistic. And if you can manage to make that happen, statistics show that you will likely live to experience many more summers on the beach and many more anniversaries than you would have otherwise.

Myth #3: I Have a Slow Metabolism

Many people think that a slow metabolism is at the root of all their problems. They gain weight just looking at food, and when they try to lose weight, their metabolism gets even slower. A tremendous number of studies have proved that the notion of a slow metabolism is misguided. According to Dr. Rudy Leibel, relative to our size, we all have the same metabolism:

> What many people don't realize is that obese people actually expend more energy than lean people do. They're bigger. They have more cells. They have more metabolic activity. But their rates of metabolism are very similar when you take their body size into consideration.

But if you think your metabolism gets slower as you're losing weight, you're actually not so far from the truth. However, it's not your metabolism slowing down, it's your body becoming more efficient at using the calories you're taking in. It's like your body has traded in its old SUV self for a shiny, new Prius, which can go much farther on every gallon of gas. The unfortunate thing about this analogy, however, is that while fuel efficiency is great for your car, the food efficiency that comes with weight loss is not great for your waistline. And it doesn't go away.

Myth #4: All It Takes Is Exercise

The millions of Americans who watch *The Biggest Loser* have witnessed countless contestants undergo miraculous transformations in their short time on the ranch by eating less and moving more—a lot more. Spending all day in the gym working out and lifting weights plays a substantial role in their rapid weight loss.

As Dr. Sam Klein, the medical director of the Washington University Weight Management Program in St. Louis puts it:

> *I cringe when I see* The Biggest Loser. *The principles proposed in that series are the antithesis of what we propose in our weight-management program, and in reputable programs around the country. The focus on physical activity as a major tool for helping people lose weight, and the extremely rigorous ordeals that patients have to go through are not something we recommend for the obese patients we treat.*

In the real world, the only people who can devote their entire day to exercise are the ones who get paid to do it—we call them professional athletes.

For most of us, it is far easier to cut down on how much we're eating than to exercise our way out of the problem. Just by drinking one of the energy drinks or protein shakes that are promoted as a way to replenish your body after a workout, you can replace in mere gulps the 100 calories you burned jogging a mile on the treadmill. Exercise also tends to increase appetite, so you might need to pay extra attention to stick to your calorie goal for the day after a session at the gym.

Clearly, exercise has its important benefits. It can help prevent heart disease, reverse diabetes, and improve a whole host of other health conditions, in addition to releasing those always-welcome endorphins that make us feel good. But the evidence of many studies shows that you shouldn't rely on exercise alone to lose weight. Where you can't succeed without it, though, is in keeping weight off, as we'll explore in detail in chapter 19.

But if the prizes you're aiming for are good health and a longer life, rather than the fleeting fame and $1 million sought by contestants on *The Biggest Loser,* changing the way you eat, along with making activity a part of your life, is the way to win.

SUCCESS STORIES

Gigi, a single mother from Nashville, works sixty hours a week in a call center to support her family. She had always believed it was selfish to spend any of the limited free time she had or over-time pay she earned on herself rather than on her daughter. But when she reached four hundred pounds at the age of forty and her doctor told her that she was beginning to show the signs of some serious chronic diseases, she had an epiphany: Not taking care of herself could mean not being there for her daughter, who had just started high school.

So Gigi kicked into high gear, completely cutting fast food from her diet and using her lunch hour at work to start walking. One year later and almost one hundred pounds lighter, she has not only transformed her own life, but she has also inspired her daughter to lose weight and helped her develop healthy habits that should last her a lifetime.

It's not just her daughter who's been inspired. Gigi's cowork-ers at the call center, many of whom struggle with their weight as well, have both supported her in her weight loss journey and even started down the same path. Gigi's not alone now in choos-ing healthy options at lunch or when she logs two miles walking around the company parking lot. It's a team effort, and everyone knows they're all healthier because of it.

17

Where to Begin

A clear set of principles guides an entire network of supervised weight-loss clinics run by hospitals around the country. One of the longest-running and foremost of these programs is based at Washington University in St. Louis and run by Dr. Sam Klein, a gastroenterologist and obesity researcher. Every patient who passes through its doors is given the evidence-based advice that we are sharing with you.

As Elana and Rhonda learned in their comparable program in New York, and as Yolanda, the inspiring woman you'll meet later in this chapter, learned in Dr. Klein's program, there are no secrets, bells, or whistles, no diets, shortcuts, or magic pills, and no getting around the hard truth that losing weight and keeping it off requires a tremendous amount of hard work. For all of them, their first step on the path to lasting weight loss was acting on their desire to attain better health by signing up for a program that could give them the tools they needed to achieve it. We're bringing the same messages and strategies to the comfort of your living room.

There's pretty much nothing in these programs that you can't do on your own, as long as you consult with your doctor. That part is really important. But there's one crucial component that you need to implement if you're going to succeed: You need to have an ongoing and reliable support system.

Cheer Tryouts

Before you do another thing, get your support system in place. Fighting the forces of fat in our world and in ourselves is no small challenge. The more people you have cheering you on, the better.

Surprisingly, when we make a commitment to make our life better, not everyone will be on board, particularly those who can't make the change for themselves. If your family or fiancé or certain friends aren't supportive, recruit others for your pep squad. Remember, though, you're far from alone. Almost 69 percent of American adults are either overweight or obese, so you are definitely not going it solo.

Feeling the Love

One of the biggest benefits of joining a group weight-loss program like Weight Watchers or Jenny (the new identity of Jenny Craig) is that it is a group of people all going on the same journey. They can provide weekly, daily, even hourly motivation. They will pump you up with success stories (even songs!) and give you a key chain or pin whenever you reach a new weight-loss milestone. But you don't have to pay for programs like these to find a group of like-minded people. Look around your local community, your Y, your place of worship, your school, and you may be surprised at how much support you can find.

Don't forget about the Internet support groups, chat rooms, and message boards dedicated to people on a weight-loss journey. Even at two in the morning when the peanut butter chocolate chip ice cream is calling your name, you can log on and get motivation from someone in Little Rock or London who understands exactly what you're going through.

A COMMITMENT TO HEALTH

The pursuit of a healthy weight is a lifelong commitment to health, and the decision to reshape your life and your health is one you should discuss with your doctor. He or she, along with other health-care professionals like registered dietitians, can make sure that the goals you set are wise, that the calories you cut are appropriate, and that the physical activity you plan to pursue is not too strenuous for your age, health, and current level of fitness.

Taking That First Step

The first step that programs like Dr. Klein's ask participants to take is to account for what they're eating and how much they're moving. The USDA reports that the average American adult (ages 19 to 50) is eating around 2,400 calories every day. If you're one of those average Americans, you are probably consuming more calories per day than you need or should. But most of us have no idea how much we're actually putting in our mouths. Just about every study that's been done to compare what people say they're eating vs what they actually consume has shown that we all drastically underestimate our intake (and overestimate how much we burn through physical activity).

You can't make a change until you know where you're starting from. Whether you use a little journal and a reference book like *The Calorie King* or keep track via an iPhone app or Web site, you need to monitor every single thing that passes your lips—food or drink—for at least a couple of weeks. It's also important to note how much activity is part of your life. This can be accomplished by clipping on a small, inexpensive pedometer to count your daily steps. At the end of those two weeks, you'll have an accurate sense of what normal means for you when it comes to eating and moving, and you can make an informed decision about the calorie cuts you'll need to make to that budget in order to lose weight sensibly. The more you're able to make activity a regular part of your day, the fewer calories you will have to give up to stay within your budget and meet your goals.

WHAT'S YOUR NUMBER?

If you want a more detailed calorie budget based on your height, weight, gender, age, and activity level, there are many online calculators that will estimate your Basal Metabolic Rate (BMR)—how many calories your body burns in its normal functioning—and help you create a plan for reaching and maintaining your weight goal. At nutrition.gov, you'll find a comprehensive list of such calculators, including links to the energy expenditure and calorie target calculators.

Setting the Right Goals

One of the things that dooms so many of us to failure is that we set goals that are too ambitious given our starting point. We're going to eat only organic food, go to the gym every day before work, cancel cable, read *War and Peace,* publish our memoirs, or climb Mount Everest. Instead, we can't even manage to eat more fruits and vegetables, walk more, cut down on TV time, read the paper, update our blogs, or take the kids camping every summer. Goals that are too lofty can prevent us from even trying to achieve them.

But if you make your goals reasonable enough that they are 100 percent attainable, there's nothing to stop you from trying. If your weight loss goal is to lose five pounds, and you do, that's something to be proud of. Now set your next goal for another five pounds. Eventually, if you do this ten times, you'll have climbed your own Mount Everest and the world will be spread out before you.

Dr. Klein would tell you that your first goal doesn't have to be about losing weight at all. Our lives are so stressful and overscheduled these days that even losing five pounds might seem out of reach. But there are steps you can take to bring that goal closer, whether it's making the time to walk fifteen minutes a day, swapping soda for water, always taking the stairs instead of the elevator, or packing a healthy lunch most days instead of eating out. If you set separate goals for each of those things, you'll get your first taste of success. We bet you'll like it—and that you'll soon be ready to take on more.

SUCCESS STORIES

Yolanda, the owner of a healthy soul food catering business, decided eighteen months ago that she needed help. While she secretly worried that her escalating weight might be affecting her health, she had trouble admitting it until her mother and sister finally intervened. It was their love that steered Yolanda to Dr. Klein and the weight-loss program at Washington University, but it was her commitment to her health and the guidance she found in the program that started her on the road to success.

Ask Yolanda how she got started, and she'll tell you that the first thing she did was to account for what she was eating and drinking—not an easy task for anyone who spends all day in a kitchen. But when she did, she had an epiphany: To her amazement, Yolanda was drinking almost 2,000 calories a day in the form of sweet tea and soda. It's probably not hard to guess what the first goal she set was: cutting out liquid calories. And she achieved it. That success helped give her the confidence to take the next step, eating a healthy breakfast every day before work. No more snacking at the stove. Yolanda did not set weight-loss goals. She set eating-behavior goals. But in the end, she lost more than 100 pounds.

Yolanda is very proud of all the weight she's lost, but as she says, "I'm even prouder of making the decision to be a healthier person."

18

Welcome to Your New Life

Once you've established a support system, logged your food intake and physical activity totals, set a calorie budget, and established some goals that are 100 percent achievable, what comes next? How do you make it through the months or years it will take to lose weight at a healthy rate and then maintain that weight loss for the rest of your life?

Remember Tim and Paul, the identical twins from Boston you met in chapter 3? Tim lost 7 percent of his body weight as part of the Diabetes Prevention Program by adding more physical activity into his life and making small changes to what he eats and drinks. These little changes were enough to reverse his prediabetes, and they have also helped him move with a spring in his step. He hits a good portion of his jump shots, his golf game has never been better, and when he goes bowling, nothing creaks, not even the floorboards.

Paul, however, who has diabetes, still weighs considerably more than Tim, doesn't get as much exercise, and recently had to add insulin to his diabetes regimen. He's come to realize the hard way that what he's been doing no longer works for him. When Tim and Paul met with Dr. David Nathan, the Harvard diabetes expert who ran the study, Paul told him, "I'm a work in progress, Doc." Dr. Nathan encouraged Paul that even now it's not too late, that with a 7 to 10 percent weight loss and an increase in physical activity he could be back off insulin and maybe even off his other diabetes medications entirely.

For Paul, it's not a matter of learning what he needs to do. He knows what he needs to do, and he's seen his identical twin brother do it. He's not lacking the knowledge; he's been lacking the commitment. Tim tells him, "You have to get up every morning and say, I'm going to do it, I will lose the 7 percent, a little bit at a time."

Paul has the support of his brother, his doctor, his family, and his friends. Now all he needs to add, he says, is the self-dedication.

Renovating Your Life

When Paul starts to make the little changes he needs to live a healthier life—or when you do—the most important thing to keep in mind is that these changes have to be sustained and become an integral part of your life. It's not a matter of starting from scratch. Think of it as the difference between building a new house and renovating the one you've got. Your motivation for renovating your life might be to spruce up your curb appeal or to fix your sagging back porch, but your contractor will tell you that if you really want to increase the value of your home, you need to update your wiring, improve your plumbing, and make sure you've got a solid foundation. Unfortunately, when it comes to our bodies, renovation is our only option—we can never build a new house or move into that model home down the block. You're going to live in this home for the rest of your life, so the time to invest in it is now.

In the rest of this chapter, we're going to give you all sorts of home improvement tips. No part of your house will be overlooked. The kitchen, the living room, the bedroom, the basement, garage, and yard. This is total lifestyle renovation.

Shop & Chop

The only place where you have total control over what you eat is in your own home. So it's crucial that you make sure your house is full of healthy food choices and that they are placed at the forefront of your pantry and refrigerator. This might require a whole new approach to where you shop, what part of the store you visit (stick to the perimeter of the supermarket, and when you duck into the aisles to grab healthy things like nuts, whole-grain pasta, and beans, don't get distracted by the junk), and how often you need to shop in order to restock fresh foods.

Studies show that when people eat a homemade meal prepared from scratch, they consume half the calories when compared to a similar meal at a restaurant. Unfortunately, many of us lack basic cooking skills, preventing us from preparing simple, quick, wholesome, delicious, and inexpensive meals for ourselves and our families. The best way to make your investment in yourself—and in your health—pay off is to invest the time in learning how to cook. You don't have to become Martha Stewart or Rachael Ray, but you can learn to cook like your grandmother did. Especially because the twenty-first century offers convenience foods that Grandma would have loved when she was young: precut vegetables and fruit, individually frozen chicken breasts, and prewashed greens. Not to mention the fact that frozen vegetables are economical, nutritious, and delicious because they have been preserved at the peak of ripeness. You can now even buy single-serving microwavable bags of frozen veggies. But make sure you avoid the varieties with added sauces and seasonings, because they often add considerable amounts of unhealthy fat, salt, or both.

Although progress is being made toward making healthier options more available where we shop and dine, the outside world will often still be a food swamp full of temptations. Make your home an island of health for you, your family, and your friends.

MISPLACED HUNGER

Denise, an attorney from Washington, D.C., noticed that her five-year-old daughter used the phrase "I'm hungry," to mean many other things, including "I'm bored," "I want attention," and most frequently, "I'm thirsty." She began replying, "No, I don't think you're hungry, I think you might be thirsty. Have a glass of water." Denise kept track, and more than 70 percent of the time, the glass of water did the trick. Her daughter would say, "You were right, Mommy. I was just thirsty."

Children don't have sophisticated communication skills, and they often have a hard time expressing what they're feeling. Instead of immediately giving in to a child's request for food, help them listen to their bodies, and explore other signals they might be receiving.

Dinnertime

The new rule about dinner? Eat together. All of you. At the table. With no TV, phones, or devices. And if you can't make it a rule every day, the more days of the week you can do this, the better everyone's health will be and the more you'll know about your kids' lives.

The National Center on Addiction and Substance Abuse at Columbia University studied the importance of the family dinner for nearly a decade. They determined that people who regularly eat with their families enjoy better health, compared with those who do not.

Kids ate more fruits and vegetables, drank less soda, and were more willing to try new foods. Parents' health improved, too, while they were modeling good behavior for their children. Kids learned how to prepare and enjoy healthy meals, solidifying good habits they could use throughout their lives. The families' diets were found to have higher-than-average amounts of many key nutrients, including calcium, iron, and fiber. And the children overall had better grades, higher self-esteem, and were less likely to use drugs because they had parents who took an active role in their daily lives.

Apparently, the family dinner table is so interesting that more than one group of researchers has studied it. A group of scientists at Harvard, led by Dr. Matt Gillman, conducted a similar study and found that 43 percent of children eat dinner with their families every day, and the number of teens who do so is even lower. They also confirmed what all parents hope is true: Children and teens who eat dinner with their families consume a healthier diet—more fruits and vegetables and less soda and fried foods.

Proper Portions

Whether at the dinner table, the breakfast counter, the office cafeteria, or the restaurant you take the whole family to on Saturday night, appropriate portion sizes have to be a constant in your life.

Far too many of us have lost any notion of what constitutes a proper portion. As we explained in chapter 9, packages of processed foods often contain multiple servings (though you might feel like you could eat a whole bag or box), and restaurant portions can be extraordinarily large.

But you have a great way to estimate serving size right in the palm of your hand. For many types of food, an almost-perfect portion is a handful, your handful. This works for just about anything: a piece of chicken, a pile of spaghetti, a scoop of ice cream, a handful of chips.

The only things you should double up on in one meal are colorful vegetables: Give yourself at least two handfuls of those.

We now live in a world where others have pre-portioned food for us, but we're paying them a premium for the service. If you have room in your calorie budget for a treat every now and then, and the treat you crave can be found in 100-calorie packs, that's a great way to limit your intake (as long as you eat just one). Or, you can achieve the same results for less money by buying a bulk bag of anything and divvying it up into individual calorie-controlled portions when you get home.

When it comes to littler hands and mouths—those of your children—the best approach is to provide them with an array of healthy foods and let them decide how much to eat based on how hungry they are.

Little Changes = Big Results

Never eat directly out of the box—of cereals, granola, crackers, or anything else. It's too hard to regulate how much you've eaten, and too easy to eat too much. Instead, pour a sensible portion (a handful) into a serving dish, and enjoy it mindfully.

Go Halfsies

The oversized restaurant portions that we explored in chapter 9 are not going the way of the dinosaur. In fact, they're a thriving species, and we need to learn how to coexist with them. Highly caloric meals dominate the menu, whether at the Olive Garden or at the finest French restaurant in town. Universal menu labeling would make it easier to pick an option that helps you stick to your calorie budget—or at least to know when you're indulging consciously and how much you'll need to compensate for it elsewhere—but we're not there yet. A simple rule to use is that, if you don't know, split anything you order in half. You could do that by setting aside half of everything on your plate, asking the server to pack up half of it to go before it even hits your table, or splitting an appetizer and an entrée with your dining partner.

The same halfsies rule can even apply to a candy bar. Yolanda, the caterer who's lost more than one hundred pounds through Dr. Klein's weight-loss program, does exactly that. She knows that depriving herself of Kit Kats makes her crazy. If she allows herself half a Kit Kat on a regular basis, she finds it easier to stick to a healthy diet the rest of the time. Of course, she saves the other half for later, right? Never. In fact, Yolanda says, "If I'm going to have a Kit Kat on my way home from work, I break it in two and throw half out before I get in the car. If I didn't, I'd be so tempted to eat it that I'd be liable to have a car accident scrounging around in my purse to find the other half."

Little Changes = Big Results

No matter what your age or size, if you find yourself in a fast-food restaurant, stick to the kids' menu. While the combo meal portions remain oversized, government and consumer pressure has led to fast-food places making improvements in their kids' meals, especially by offering healthier options. It might seem smaller than you're used to, but one kids' meal is definitely enough calories, and it'll still satisfy your craving. You may keep the toy.

Fighting the Urge to Splurge

No matter how you stock your cupboards and your fridge, unless you grow all your own food, homeschool your kids, and never leave the house, it's nearly impossible for you and your family to escape all temptations. Even at the farmers' market, when you're virtuously shopping for vegetables, you need to use your smarts to avoid the siren call of the spelt-crust apple turnover or the seven-grain cheese bread. And if you find yourself near the food court at the mall or passing the vending machine on your way to your desk from the stairwell, the delicious, calorie-dense concoctions that call out to you will be that much harder to resist.

Moving about in our world without succumbing to all those temptations requires us to exert an enormous amount of self-control. Remember the role of your prefrontal cortex, the executive center of your brain that we told you about in chapter 7? This is where it comes into play. The evolutionarily ancient core of our brain knows only to say yes when it comes to food. The food industry knows this, and spends billions of dollars to make food irresistibly appealing. Clearly, it's getting a return on its investment, because far too many of us are saying yes far too often. Either executive function isn't powerful enough, or the ancient pulls are too strong.

Plan Ahead

The same way someone with severe allergies shouldn't leave the house without an EpiPen, or someone with asthma doesn't go out without an inhaler, people struggling with their weight should not venture into the world unarmed. It's a lot harder to resist temptation if your stomach is growling. Hunger is uncomfortable for a reason. It's a signal that you need to eat. If you always travel with your own supply of healthy snacks, though, you're in control, not your stomach. Keep snacks like fruit, nuts, or baby carrots in your car, your briefcase or purse, your desk, or your teenager's backpack, so that you and your kids don't undo all of your hard work with a stop at the newsstand or a trip to the vending machine.

In addition to always having a supply of healthy snacks on hand, another tactic is to plan ahead for those times when the food you've grown up loving is available in abundance: during holidays, at parties, and at other meaningful events, such as weddings or anniversary celebrations. The cultural association between good times and food is imprinted on us as early as our first birthday, not to mention our first Thanksgiving. And most of us don't want to feel different or call attention to ourselves because we are now eating less. If you don't leave room in your budget for celebrating holidays around a dinner table or joining your kids in an occasional ice cream cone, it's going to be hard to make these new habits work for you in the long run.

Going to these events hungry will inevitably weaken your resolve. Instead, eat a healthy snack before heading to Aunt Sally's July Fourth barbecue. You'll be less hungry heading in and therefore better prepared to stick to just one hot dog and turn down a second helping of her famous macaroni salad. When faced with a buffet or cocktail hour, try to make your portion sizes resemble sample sizes. This will satisfy your brain's desire to graze and consume the widest variety of food possible without having to loosen your belt by the end of the night.

And how to handle the holiday season, when special occasions seem to come along every night? A recent study shows that people who walk or run regularly are less likely to gain weight, even when they overindulge around the holidays. And the more miles you walk or run, the less likely you are to look in the mirror on the first of the year and fall right back into the old trap of New Year's resolutions.

WALK 100 MILES

Last spring, Mayor Karl Dean of Nashville, Tennessee, invited the people of Nashville to join him in making physical activity a regular and fun part of their lives by walking one hundred miles in three months. The mayor wanted Nashvillians to get healthier while at the same time discovering the city's dozens of parks and hundreds of miles of new greenways.

The mayor's challenge was a great success. Thousands of people signed up online to log their miles, walk on their own, and join him every week. Carol, a fifty-year-old artist, was among them. She had been attempting to lose weight for years and had tried many different programs, from Weight Watchers to Spark-People. She understood the changes she needed to make to her diet and lifestyle, and regularly offered support to—and received it from—others who understood her struggle. Despite this, Carol felt she had hit a wall. She had lost some weight initially, but just couldn't get past a plateau.

There was one thing left she hadn't tried: regular physical activity. Even the notion of going for a walk was alien to her. But Mayor Dean inspired her and her husband, Bill. One month into the challenge, they had both already walked more than one hundred miles, and were starting to see the benefits. By the summer, hundreds of miles later, Carol had left her plateau far behind.

Get Moving

Just as your new relationship to food is of the "till death do us part" variety, so must be your relationship to moving your body. And we're not going to call it exercise. You don't have to sweat it out at the gym, run around the high school track, or join a soccer league (though all of those are great). You just need to move more. Even walking counts. But to make it count, you have to do it often and go farther than the end of your block. Biking, swimming, dancing, yoga, skiing—these are all great options for you to weave into your life. And the more you pepper the mix with different activities, the spicier your life will be.

If helping your kids with their homework or keeping up with your own night school schedule doesn't leave you with half an hour for an evening stroll, your only option is to look closely at your day and be creative about any opportunity for incorporating some activity into it. Park ten or fifteen minutes from your office and walk the rest of the way. If it's raining, drive all the way to work, but use those ten or fifteen minutes to walk up and down the stairs a few times. Once you make this part of your life, anything that gets in the way of physical activity will come to feel like an intrusion. You'll begin to look forward to your walks not just for their health benefits, but for their mind-clearing effects. When else do you have time to be alone and think?

Tame the Tube Time

Another crucial step to take if you're going to succeed at losing weight and keeping it off? Minimize your TV and computer time. If you watch fewer cooking shows and ball games, you might suddenly find the inspiration to become a gourmet chef or turn into a backyard quarterback.

Move the TV out of your bedroom. Impose limits on how much TV your kids can watch. You might even ask them to earn their screen time with physical activity.

Research has shown that the connection between weight gain and screen time isn't completely attributed to spending all that time sitting instead of moving. The barrage of food commercials on TV definitely does not help. To avoid them, watch your favorite TV series on demand, record them and fast-forward through all the commercials when you watch later, wait until they come out on DVD, or subscribe to a pay cable network, like HBO, that doesn't have commercials.

The Power of Sleep

By now you should know by heart that losing weight is about eating less and moving more. But here's something new—emerging research is indicating that you can also complement these efforts throughout the day by getting more good sleep at night. Unfortunately, we are becoming a sleep-deprived nation. Daily sleep duration among adults has gone down by one to two hours in the past forty years, and the number of us getting less than seven hours has doubled. Even worse, this trend seems to be affecting all ages.

Little Changes = Big Results

It seems that Benjamin Franklin might have been right about the importance of being "early to bed, early to rise." Some researchers have found that people who go to bed later and get up later not only consume more calories after 8 P.M., but also consume more total calories throughout the day. You might consider trying to go to bed earlier and getting up earlier if you want to be "healthy and wise." (Wealthy we can't promise.)

How much sleep do you need? There's no magic number, but the National Sleep Foundation gives us a "rule of thumb" number that experts agree with. Adults should get between 7.5 and 9 hours a night, while teenagers need about 9 hours, grade-school kids 10 to 11, preschoolers 11 to 13, infants 14 to 15, and newborns 12 to 18.

And quality matters. Light, restless, or interrupted sleep is just as detrimental to your body as too little sleep. Some tips for getting a good night's sleep:
- Don't drink any liquids after 8 P.M.
- Stop drinking caffeine six hours before bedtime.
- Quit any stressful or work activity two hours before bedtime.
- Remove TV or game systems from bedrooms.

Researchers have long known about the restorative powers of sleep but have only recently begun to produce evidence that points to short sleep duration as a risk factor for obesity. Simply put, scientists have discovered that, when you slumber, your brain secretes powerful metabolism-regulating hormones. When you don't get enough sleep, there is an immediate, measurable, detrimental effect on glucose metabolism; a decrease in the production of leptin, the hormone that tells your brain you have enough fat stores; and an increase in the appetite-stimulating hormone, ghrelin.

The day after you don't get enough sleep, your body is hungrier, less easily satisfied, and doesn't process glucose as well.

Just how bad is it? A study of people who slept four hours a night for two nights compared to when they slept ten hours for two nights found that when they got less sleep, their ghrelin-to-leptin ratio increased by more than 70 percent, their overall hunger increased 23 percent, and their craving for carbs went up more than 30 percent. A similar study of healthy young men found that just two nights of restricted sleep lowered their glucose tolerance by 40 percent, putting them on a level with prediabetic elderly people.

ROCK-A-BYE BABY

Pediatric researchers are beginning to think that establishing a good sleep routine from birth is an important factor in a child's future weight. Doctors at Harvard Medical School discovered that infants and toddlers who slept less than twelve hours a night were twice as likely to be overweight by preschool than those who got more than twelve hours of sleep. Even if you have a fussy sleeper or a natural night owl, it's never too late to get your kids into a better sleep pattern.

19

How to Keep It Off

All the people you've met throughout the pages of this book—Tim and Paul, Elana and Rhonda, Tom, Gigi, Yolanda, and Carol—have a single thing in common: Each of them reached a point, after years of carrying too much weight, when they realized that the way they were living their lives no longer worked for them. They could no longer ignore the health consequences of eating too much, moving too little, and gaining too much weight.

Like the rest of us, their weight gain was gradual, a few additional pounds each year going by unnoticed. They buckled their belts in the next notch, felt their wedding bands getting tighter, and were a little more winded at the top of the stairs. That second helping of Aunt Millie's lasagna, a night spent sprawled on the couch watching an old movie with the family, and the regular trip to the Waffle House on Sundays after church: These were the small things they all took pleasure in. In our busy lives, with jobs to go to, children to raise, bills to pay, and not enough time, we have to take pleasure where we can.

Gigi, for example, thought that the overtime pay she earned was the best way she had to invest in her daughter's future. It wasn't until her doctor told her that her weight would likely cut her life short that she was able to put herself and her health before her paycheck and lose more than a hundred pounds.

For Tim, who was thirty pounds or so overweight, it wasn't until his identical twin, Paul, developed diabetes that he began to worry and asked his doctor about his own risk. After his blood work showed that he was prediabetic, he lost 7 percent of his body weight—just fourteen pounds—and has beaten the 95 percent odds that the identical twin of someone with diabetes will also develop the disease.

But many of these weight-loss success stories did not start out that way. Almost everyone we've introduced you to tried countless diets and always regained any weight they lost. Every diet can promise that you'll lose weight, because it's true. If you deprive yourself for a while, you will lose weight, but once you do and you return to eating the way you used to, the weight will follow you. There are few things more unnatural for our species than to deliberately deprive ourselves of food.

The false premise is that diets can wipe the slate clean, that our new slimmer bodies retain no memory of their previous, larger selves. The unfortunate truth is that our bodies never forget. When we lose weight, our bodies work to maintain their former status quo, and it's very difficult for our brain to ignore those signals. If we take a short-term approach to weight loss, failure is almost inevitable. And each time our weight yo-yos, our body strengthens its defenses. The people profiled here did not succeed until they finally took control of their lives and changed their lifestyle.

And that's exactly what you need to do, too. There's a reason the previous chapter was called "Welcome to Your New Life," and it's because that's what this is. It's like the difference between paying the minimum on your credit card bill each month and paying off what you owe. If you take only a short-term approach, you're never going to be unburdened. When it comes to your weight, your best chance of finding freedom is to realize that your life isn't working for you and to change the way you live it.

Changing the way you live your life is not easy. It's really hard to lose weight, and as we're sure you've understood by now, it's going to be harder still to keep it off. Even if you succeed at achieving a healthy weight, you will have to stay vigilant in your efforts to maintain it. Remember the unfair truth you learned from our imaginary friends Ellen and Kate in chapter 6? Maintaining your new weight is going to be harder for you than for someone who has always been at that weight.

Having to watch your weight is no different from dealing with any other health condition that must be monitored continuously. If you have high blood pressure, the doctor isn't going to tell you to bring it down for six months, and then do whatever you want. People with diabetes, even when they have it under control, still have to manage it forever.

It may not seem fair. But that's life.

Being healthy isn't a temporary state of being. It's a lifelong benefit. Managing your weight, watching what you eat, staying active, and tuning out all the messages and cues that test your resolve will now and forever be a part of your daily life—but it will also help you have a happy, healthy, and longer one.

Weight Winners

The National Weight Control Registry has been tracking more than five thousand people who have lost significant amounts of weight and kept it off for a long time. The average participant has lost sixty-six pounds and kept it off for five and a half years, but weight losses range from thirty to three hundred pounds, and many participants have kept it off for decades. Roughly half the people in the registry lost their weight as part of a program like Weight Watchers or a medically supervised program like the ones in which Elana, Rhonda, and Yolanda enrolled, but 45 percent of them say they did it all on their own. In surveying their behaviors, the researchers discovered that almost all the successful "losers" shared a few important behaviors:

- 62 percent watch fewer than ten hours of TV a week
- 78 percent weigh themselves at least once a week, many daily
- 78 percent eat breakfast every day
- 90 percent exercise about one hour a day on average
- 98 percent continue to eat a healthier diet
- 100 percent say their quality of life is higher

Too Big to Fix?

As a nation, we have a huge obesity problem. But America has so far never faced a problem that was too big to fix.

Sixty years ago, people littered with impunity, seat belts weren't an option (let alone the law), and even Santa Claus smoked. Collectively or working together, we managed to recognize those problems and reverse those trends, and to raise a new generation that recycles, buckles up, and sees smoking as a serious health risk.

If small changes in the way we live our lives are responsible for our weight gain, they are likely enough to help us turn it around for ourselves.

The first step you can take is to arm yourself with the right knowledge. We hope you feel that this book has given you what you need to begin. Own your new life. Enjoy it. And share your joy with those around you—your family, your friends, and your community.

But what we haven't told you is that even if millions of overweight people made those little changes, it probably wouldn't be enough to reverse the curve and turn the obesity epidemic around. For every pound you lose, someone else is probably gaining one. And, sadly, the statistics are telling us that that person could very well be a child.

We need to work together as a nation to make some big changes to the systems that govern the food we grow; the economies that drive the food we manufacture, market, and serve; the policies that regulate what we market and serve, particularly to kids; the values we place on the overall quality of the schools to which we send our children; the design of our communities, parks, and roads so they promote health; and the perspective of our health-care system so that it's focused on preventing illness from happening, rather than just treating it once it develops.

In order to solve America's obesity crisis, we all need to be involved. For ourselves, for our kids, and for the future of our country. The challenges presented by the obesity epidemic are different from the ones posed by cancer, HIV, addiction, or Alzheimer's. We've seen those as wars we have to fight, and we've devoted billions of dollars to those battles. But obesity is not only a disease; it's also a condition of our modern lifestyle. In fact, a closer comparison is probably to global warming.

When Henry Ford introduced the Model T to America, he thought he was giving us a new, faster means of transportation that would make life easier and better for all of us. And he did. But the billions of pounds of carbon emissions we're dealing with today are the unintended consequences of progress. The same is true of the obesity epidemic. We learned how to double and triple our agricultural yields, enabling us to feed not just our country, but also much of the world; processed the crops we grow into an infinite array of delicious foods; constructed suburbs and superhighways and shopping malls; invented everything from vacuum cleaners and microwaves to television, computers, and iPads. The obesity epidemic developed concurrently with all those improvements in our lifestyle. And who would choose to go back to a time where we lived without these things?

But until we embrace a different view of the *purpose* of modern life, and begin to value health as much as convenience, comfort, and cost, not much is going to change. It's time for America to make the healthy choice the easy choice—instead of the hard, inconvenient, or more expensive one.

Obesity is a political issue, an economic issue, a social issue, a health issue, and a personal issue. Every reader of this book has the capacity to bring about change in at least one of those areas. You've made the decision to start with yourself. You know what you have to do. You are not alone. And you can do it.

Afterword:
Dialing Back the
Weight of the Nation

Mark Twain famously observed, "It's easy to quit smoking. I've done it hundreds of times." The irony behind Twain's observation applies to many of us who have lost more pounds than we weigh over the course of a lifetime. It is one thing to slim down to a healthier weight, quite another to keep off the extra pounds. I admire those who manage to maintain a lifetime of healthy weight. Most of us do not.

Biology and environment conspire against us. Relatively inexpensive, abundant, appealing high-calorie foods beckon us, and we are programmed to consume more calories than we require to meet our bodily needs. We have configured our work and living conditions to reduce physical exertion. Even manual labor often demands less than in earlier days: control paddles replace levers on heavy equipment, leaf and snow blowers do the job of rakes and shovels. At home, televisions and computer monitors keep us glued to our seats. We have replaced walking with an automotive culture and reduced daily time for active play and physical education. Our children take the bus rather than walk or bike to school, burning diesel fuel instead of calories.

The fault lies not in our stars. It is right here with us on earth, within us and around us. Of course, we can do more for ourselves: becoming aware and wary of the empty calories in sugary soft drinks and the fatty calories hidden in many foods, being thoughtful about portion size, and adopting the practice of mindful eating. The problem of overweight and obesity, however, is not only a problem of individuals—it is a social phenomenon that expresses itself in millions of Americans. When the majority of us have become overweight or obese, and more so with every passing year, solving the problem will demand more than isolated, individual effort to lose weight.

If we are going to dial back the weight of the nation, we will need to act together—as families, communities, and a nation—to make the right individual choices easier, cheaper, more satisfying, and more convenient. We need to engage government at all levels and private enterprise to create the conditions where more of us can attain and maintain a healthy weight for a lifetime. The first lady, Michelle Obama, is a grand champion of the cause. Companies like Walmart, in adopting healthier standards for its branded foods and lowering prices on fresh fruit and vegetables, set a fine example. This book, the HBO documentary series of the same name, and the companion report from the Institute of Medicine, *Accelerating Progress in Obesity Prevention*, all point the way. Now it is simply up to us to act in our own best interests.

The book you have finished is not a diet book. It contains no magical recipes and reveals no secrets to weight loss. Oddly enough, however, if we heed its message, this could be the last diet book you will ever need.

—Harvey V. Fineberg, M.D., Ph.D.
President, Institute of Medicine

Tips for Healthy Eating While Watching Calories

Whether you're trying to lose weight, maintaining a weight loss, or protecting yourself from gaining too much to begin with, one of the easiest ways to stay within your calorie budget is to consume a healthy diet full of whole, nutrient-rich foods whenever possible. Try to ensure you eat a variety of vegetables and fruits, lean proteins, whole grains, and low-fat and fat-free dairy products, while reducing consumption of sugar-sweetened beverages. As Rhonda, Elana's weight-loss partner profiled in chapter 6, would tell you, the best way to maximize the amount of food you can take in without busting your calorie budget is to "eat lots of salad and vegetables, sauce on the side, always on the side." Choosing to eat a variety of bright, colorful vegetables will keep your palate entertained and fill you up with fiber so you don't feel like you're running on empty just because you've cut back on your calories.

We've got lots of tips in store for you below, but if you finish and are still hungry for more, check out ChooseMyPlate.gov and the Weight-control Information Network (http://win.niddk.nih.gov).

Foods for a Healthy Lifestyle

+ Lean meat, poultry, and seafood
+ Lots of vegetables
+ Lots of fruit
+ Whole grains
+ Beans, peas, eggs, and nuts and seeds
+ Low-fat and fat-free dairy or other calcium-rich foods
+ Healthy oils such as olive, canola, or walnut

Homemade Treats

You can allow yourself sweets and treats in moderation, but to keep the portion reasonable and avoid extra fat and sugar, make them yourself. Anything you can find premixed in a box—cakes, cookies, pancakes, brownies—you can usually make at home for less money, in just a little more time, with ingredients you likely already have in your pantry. And you'll eliminate from your diet those trans fats and hidden sugars your body just doesn't need. You're also likely to bake a bit less often when you're doing all the work yourself.

Three great tips: Freeze half the batch or give it away to a neighbor, so you don't have too much lying around; make only a half batch to begin with; and use healthier substitutions wherever you can, for instance, unsweetened applesauce for vegetable oil in baked goods.

Perfect Portions

The research of psychologist Dr. Brian Wansink, who runs the Cornell University Food and Brand Lab, shows that we can easily be tricked into eating more than we should. In one of his experiments, he served subjects soup from bowls that were constantly being refilled by a hidden tube—and the subjects kept on eating until they had consumed a very large amount of soup. What we can learn from this is that we can also trick ourselves into eating less. Replace your dinner plate with a salad plate, and the smaller portion you dish out won't seem nearly so small. Replace your standard glassware with juice glasses, and you'll notice the same thing about how much you're drinking: A small serving seems bigger when it's presented in a small glass.

What Not to Eat

In a perfect world, we would eat only fresh food grown on the farm in our backyard. But we live in a far-from-perfect world. And most of us live far from the farm. Therefore, we have to make the most of our shopping options.

As long as you're eating an appropriate amount of calories for your weight goals, there's nothing you absolutely shouldn't ever eat (except maybe trans fats). No one ever became obese from one meal. The important thing is that you recognize the difference between healthy foods and their unhealthy counterparts and choose the healthy option as frequently as you can.

Don't Buy Into Bogus Claims

When looking for healthy food in the grocery store, you can almost ignore the front of the boxes entirely. As we've mentioned earlier, "healthier" doesn't mean healthy; "less fat" doesn't mean an appropriate amount of fat.

Check out the nutrition label, avoid anything with industrially produced trans fat, and count the ingredients. Too many (or too many you can't pronounce), and it's time to reconsider that box.

There's No Such Thing as a Free Lunch

Oil is a fat. There's no way it can be "fat-free." Sugar has calories. Food scientists can develop sugar substitutes that are "calorie-free," but they are still made of something. And do most of us really need them? Or at least do we need to use a lot of them?

The lesson learned: Stick to food that's as close to its natural state as possible. Sugar, olive oil, and small amounts of butter have been used safely for thousands of years, but use them sparingly.

Secret Sugars

The American Heart Association recommends that women eat no more than 100 calories from added sugars a day; that's about six teaspoons or 25 grams. For men, the recommendation is no more than 150 calories from added sugars, which is about 38 grams or nine teaspoons. It's obvious that Froot Loops and candy bars have added sugar, but plenty of other everyday foods have added sugars you wouldn't expect, including the following:

- Spaghetti sauce: Some brands have as much as three teaspoons of sugar per half cup.
- Low-fat salad dressing: Fat that is removed is often replaced with sugar.
- Bagels: Especially fruit, cinnamon, or honey-flavored ones can have two teaspoons or more per bagel.
- Fruit-flavored yogurt: There are many health benefits of yogurt, but the added sugar in many yogurts may outweigh the good effects.
- Ketchup: A ¼ cup—4 tablespoons—gives you the same amount of sugar as ⅓ of a can of soda.

Sweet by Any Other Name

Sugar doesn't always announce itself as "sugar" on the ingredient list. These are some of its common pseudonyms:

agave nectar
brown sugar
cane crystals

cane sugar

corn sugar

corn sweetener

corn syrup

crystalline fructose

dextrose

evaporated cane juice

fructose

fruit juice concentrates

glucose

high-fructose corn syrup

honey

invert sugar

lactose

maltose

malt syrup

molasses

sucrose

syrup

Skip the Bakery and Coffee Shop Desserts

There's no quicker way to ruin a healthy lunch or your virtuous unsweetened coffee with skim milk than to cave to the temptation to add a tiny baked treat. There's nothing tiny about the fat and calories in most of the baked goods you buy at a bakery, coffee shop, restaurant, or supermarket. Imagine you kept your lunch low-calorie and low-fat by filling up on a bowl of low-fat chicken soup at Panera with just 120 calories and 1.5 grams of fat. You included the French baguette for dipping, which added 150 calories with just 1 gram of fat. But add the thin, rather harmless-looking chocolate chip cookie, and you'll add 440 calories and 23 grams of fat (14 grams of it saturated) to your budget.

Even the minis and "bite-sized" are suspect. Most tiny treats at Starbucks pack 200 calories into just two bites!

Skip the pastries and wait twenty minutes, and the craving will probably have passed—if not, have a piece of sweet, ripe fruit!

What to Drink

Learning to live without sugary beverages in a world where $948 million is spent to market them each year is no easy task. Treat yourself to the best coffee you can afford, so you don't have to hide the taste with cream and sugar. Experiment with new and exotic teas. Grow your own mint on a sunny windowsill and use it to dress up your water and tea, or add a wedge of lemon or lime.

And how can you change your kids' drinking habits? Introduce your kids to that fancy metal contraption called a drinking fountain. When they're thirsty, the first thing you offer them should be cold, good-tasting water. If you do give them juice, first make sure it's 100-percent fruit juice and then dilute it with water or seltzer. They'll still get the sweetness with half the sugar.

You can cut your calorie intake instantly without missing a bite of food if you cut out your high-calorie (low-nutrient) drinks. Here's to your health:

Water

Water, water, water. Plain water. Sparkling water. Water with a dash of 100-percent fruit juice. Water with a slice of lemon, lime, cucumber, or watermelon.

Tea

Drink it without added cream or sugar. Add a little skim milk if you like it lighter. Drink it hot, or pour it over ice and drink it cold.

Coffee

All the same rules for tea apply to coffee: It's best black or with skim milk. And stick to a good old cup of joe—skip the frothy mixes, whipped cream, and sprinkled toppings.

Skim Milk and Soy Milk

Packed with calcium and vitamin D. Choose nonfat or low-fat (1 percent) milk, including soy, rice, or almond beverages, fortified with calcium and vitamins A and D.

Fruit or Vegetable Juice

Only 100 percent juice. But it's important to get the majority of your fruit and veggie servings from whole fruit or veggies instead of from juice. For vegetable juices, look for low-sodium varieties.

WHAT ABOUT DIET SODA?

The jury is still out on diet soda. If you must get your soda fix, it's definitely a better option than regular soda, but researchers believe that it might not be entirely benign. And we're not just talking about the role of artificial sweeteners. There is no evidence to support claims that they might actually be inherently harmful. However, some scientists hypothesize that, because over the course of human evolution, our ancestors never encountered the taste of sweetness without a load of calories, our bodies do not know how to handle the artificial sweeteners in diet sodas and other no-calorie products. When we consume something sweet, our body expects a sugar rush and releases insulin into the bloodstream in anticipation of the need to deal with it. These researchers theorize that when we drink a diet soda, we don't actually experience that influx of sugar. But the insulin sticks around, making us hungry and increasing our consumption over the course of the day. In the end, drinking soda, whether regular or diet, may increase our caloric intake.

What Not to Drink

It's worth repeating: Don't drink your meals—or even your snacks. Nothing is entirely forbidden, but the less of this stuff you drink, the better you'll feel (and look). Keep in mind that this list is not exhaustive. With few exceptions (such as skim or low-fat milk), most drinks with calories are something you should consume infrequently and in small amounts. That goes for alcohol, too!

Soda

One twelve-ounce can of soda has about eight teaspoons of added sugar, usually in the form of high-fructose corn syrup.

Energy Drinks

Soda on steroids, with high amounts of added sugar and caffeine. Beware.

Flavored Water

There are some no-calorie vitamin waters, but there are just as many that contain plenty of added sugar. If you want to flavor your water, use real fruit (vitamins included for free).

Sweetened Tea and Lemonade

Usually just as caloric as soda but without the carbonation. Add a strawberry or raspberry flavoring, and you'll bump up the calories by as much as 30 percent.

Ices, Slushies, Freezes, and Chillers

Often highly caloric, often laden with sugary syrup. Soda-flavored varieties even kick in some caffeine.

Fruit-Flavored Drinks

Marketed to kids, these brightly hued drinks are practically the equivalent of colored sugar water.

Fruit Smoothies

Often a source of added sugars and even fats. Think of it as a colorful milk shake. A fruit smoothie may have hundreds more calories than you bargained for. A "low-fat" smoothie can contain as much as 15 grams of fat, more than a Snickers bar.

Blended, Creamy Coffee Drinks

If you order mindlessly at the coffee counter, you could find yourself with a cup containing 500 calories with 15 grams of saturated fat and 75 grams of sugar.

Blended, Creamy, Frozen Coffee Drinks

Even worse because ice cream is added into the mix. Dairy Queen's twenty-four-ounce Caramel MooLatté has 870 calories, 19 grams of saturated fat, 1 gram of trans fat, and 112 grams of sugar.

Bottled Coffee Drinks

Just as bad as blended, creamy coffees, but without the ability to substitute low-fat milk as you can when custom-ordering at the coffee shop.

Hot Chocolate

A twenty-ounce Starbucks Peppermint Hot Chocolate (with whole milk and whipped cream) comes with more than 500 calories, 14 grams of saturated fat, and 79 grams of sugar.

Shakes and Floats

If you're craving ice cream, have just a single ½-cup scoop. A milkshake will often give you the equivalent of six or more scoops and can run up to 1,000 calories with 25 grams of saturated fat, 1.5 grams of trans fats, and more than 120 grams of sugar. Ditto on the root beer float.

Tips for Active Living

Just as healthy eating is crucial for sticking to your calorie budget in order to prevent weight gain, maintain a weight loss, or lose weight, adopting an active lifestyle also plays an important role. And we don't just mean exercise. Physical activity is any form of body movement that uses energy. Since it causes the body to use more calories, you can see how physical activity helps contribute to calorie deficit (for weight loss) or calorie balance (for weight maintenance).

Even if you are already at a healthy weight, physical activity has a great deal of health benefits. For example, strong evidence shows that it can help lower the risk of heart disease, stroke, type 2 diabetes, high blood pressure, and colon and breast cancers; prevent falls; reduce depression; and improve cognitive function in older adults. It also leads to the release of endorphins that make us feel good—you could say it provides a natural high. Before you fall back on all those excuses for why you don't have the time, money, or equipment to engage in regular physical activity, consider the kind of activities and time investments that count toward achieving these recommendations—they might not be as tough as you expect.

Physical Activity Guidelines for Americans

In 2008, the U.S. Department of Health and Human Services released the first set of Physical Activity Guidelines for Americans. We'll give you highlights of the recommendations for adults ages 18 to 64 here, but for the full version (which includes recommendations for children, older adults, and adults with disabilities) go to health.gov/paguidelines. To receive the greatest health benefits, adults should do moderate-intensity aerobic activities—those that make your heart beat faster and can make your heart, lungs, and blood vessels stronger and more fit—for at least 150 minutes (2 hours, 30 minutes) per week. If you step it up a notch to vigorous aerobic activity, a mere 75 minutes per week will do the trick. See the lists below to understand the difference between the two. There's no harm in doing a combination of the two, and it's best to spread your activity over three or more days of the week. The more time you spend being physically active, the more benefits you gain.

How do you know how intense your activity is? A good rule of thumb is that if you can talk but not sing while doing it, it is moderate activity, whereas during vigorous activity you shouldn't be able to say more than a few words without stopping to catch your breath.

Moderate Activities

- Ballroom and line dancing
- Biking on level ground or with few hills
- Canoeing
- General gardening (raking, trimming shrubs)
- Sports where you catch and throw (baseball, softball, volleyball)
- Tennis (doubles)
- Using a manual wheelchair

- Using hand cyclers—also called ergometers
- Walking briskly
- Water aerobics

Vigorous Activities

- Aerobic dance
- Biking faster than 10 miles per hour
- Fast dancing
- Heavy gardening (digging, hoeing)
- Hiking uphill
- Jumping rope
- Martial arts (such as karate)
- Race walking, jogging, or running
- Sports with a lot of running (basketball, hockey, soccer)
- Swimming fast or swimming laps
- Tennis (singles)

Two and a half hours of moderate activity per week can be broken down into 30 minutes, five times a week. Don't think you can round up an extra half hour to be active? You're in luck. Bouts of 10 or 15 minutes count, too, as long as they add up to 30 at the end of the day. Take a brisk stroll with the dog before you leave for work, park a little farther from your office and power-walk across the parking lot, and rake some leaves after dinner, and you've easily accumulated at least 30 minutes. And if you're going for vigorous activity, you can get similar results in half the time—15 minutes, five days a week.

If you've been inactive for a long time and don't think you can do a total of 30 minutes of activity in a day, then start with a smaller amount and gradually increase the intensity and duration of activity. Some activity is definitely better than none. Walking is a great first step to be active. And besides investing in a sturdy pair of walking shoes, it's one of the cheapest and easiest forms of activity. When it's cold outside, you can head over to the mall and do some laps there if you don't want to face the elements.

In addition to aerobic activities, strengthening activities—those that make your muscles work harder than usual—are important for reaping the maximum health benefits. Aim to do these kinds of activities at least two days per week, working the major muscle groups: legs, hips, back, chest, stomach, shoulders, and arms. Exercises for each muscle group should be repeated 8 to 12 times per session. Examples include lifting weights, push-ups, sit-ups, or working with resistance bands (long, wide, rubber strips that stretch). You don't have to invest in fancy equipment or a gym membership—you can "pump iron" with common grocery items like soup cans, bags of rice, or water bottles instead of dumbbells.

Have It Your Way

You'll be more likely to stick to a regular physical activity routine if you customize it to your lifestyle and interests. Here are some other tips for succeeding in maintaining a physically active lifestyle:

- Choose activities that you like and that fit into your life.
- Find the time that works best for you.
- Enlist friends and family to be active with you—for example, find a walking buddy or help your neighbor with yard work.
- Set goals, and monitor your progress toward them. Once you've achieved them, set more ambitious goals.

It's also a good idea to discuss any proposed changes to your activity level with your doctor. He or she can help ensure you ease into an active lifestyle and don't take on too much at once.

Healthy Pregnancy, Healthy Baby

If you are thinking about becoming pregnant, this is an important section of the book for you to read. We tucked it back here at the end because it doesn't apply to everyone. But if you are currently expecting, or expect to be at some point, the advice we're about to give you is important not only for ensuring you have a healthy pregnancy but also for establishing a healthy future for your child.

Parenthood begins before the first trimester. The decisions you make, both before getting pregnant and between conception and delivery, help set the stage for a healthy pregnancy and a healthy baby. The weight at which you enter a pregnancy and how many pounds you gain during it, as well as your habits during pregnancy—what you eat and drink, how much activity you get—are important for both your health and that of your child. In fact, emerging evidence suggests these factors can help set your child on a healthy course for life. And we know that women who are at a higher weight going into a pregnancy have a greater chance of having children who are likely to be obese. The issues of weight and weight gain during pregnancy are serious ones.

Eating for 1.2

When the IOM released its previous set of guidelines for weight gain during pregnancy in 1990, overweight and obese women made up a significantly smaller portion of the population than they do today. For years, doctors had worried that many women, out of concern for their weight, would not eat enough to nourish the fetus and allow it to develop normally. A low pre-pregnancy weight is one of the predictors of adverse outcomes during pregnancy, and the 1990 guidelines reflected that. This notion is echoed in popular culture as the common belief that, when you're pregnant, you can eat for two. Pregnancy is the one time in many women's lives when they don't feel guilty about ordering that ice cream sundae or indulging at a buffet. Pregnant women are humored when they have weird food cravings, at any hour, and often allow themselves frequent overindulgences. But they shouldn't.

The obesity epidemic has changed things. Today, according to the CDC, there are 62 million American women of childbearing age, and nearly 40 million of them are overweight or obese. IOM reexamined its guidelines and in May 2009 released new recommendations, which for the first time include a specific and relatively narrow range of recommended gain for obese women, with a strict upper limit.

Here are the current IOM guidelines for pregnancy weight gain, based on your BMI before becoming pregnant (unless you're expecting multiples, in which case, the recommended weight gain goes up a bit):

Underweight (BMI < 18.5): Gain 28 to 40 pounds
Healthy weight (BMI 18.5 to 24.9): Gain 25 to 35 pounds
Overweight (BMI 25 to 29.9): Gain 15 to 25 pounds
Obese (BMI ≥ 30): Gain 11 to 20 pounds

Harvard researcher Dr. Matt Gillman, who served on the IOM committee responsible for the new guidelines, hopes that they inspire women to change how they think about weight gain during pregnancy. "Instead of eating for two, what if they thought about eating for 1.2?" And in the first trimester, just keep eating for one, then add about 350 extra calories per day for the rest of the pregnancy. That shift in perspective might go a long way toward helping women prevent the pregnancy pounds from piling on.

OFF TO A GOOD START

As important as it is to avoid gaining excess weight during pregnancy, it's even more crucial to start out at a healthy weight. If you are currently overweight or obese, you might want to pursue prenatal counseling before trying to conceive. Bring it up with your doctor, and say that you are thinking about getting pregnant but wonder if your weight, diet, and exercise habits have you prepared for carrying a healthy baby. He or she can help you figure out whether you should try to lose some weight before giving it a go, and can refer you to another health-care provider, such as a registered dietitian, to develop a diet and physical activity plan.

Complications

Overweight and obesity may be partly responsible for the record-high rates of Caesarean sections that we're currently witnessing, and may also contribute to poor birth outcomes. As a woman's BMI rises, so does the percentage of surgical births, climbing from 11 percent in women who are at a healthy weight to 18 percent in overweight women, 25 percent among obese women, and 43 percent among morbidly obese women. In addition to stillbirth, which is twice as likely, and premature delivery, obese women also face an increased risk of gestational diabetes, high blood pressure during pregnancy (preeclampsia), hemorrhage, blood clots, strokes, and complications from anesthesia.

LOSING THOSE PREGNANCY POUNDS

Many women can trace their struggles with weight back to their pregnancy: "I never had a problem until after I had Maddy. But I just wasn't able to shake that weight. My body has never been the same."

Baby weight can be especially hard to shake because of the lack of sleep and increased demands on our time that inevitably follow the birth of a baby and never really disappear. But it's especially important to make every effort to lose it, especially if you're thinking about having another. Don't let the excess pounds you put on during your first pregnancy doom you to a heavier and more difficult subsequent one.

One of the best ways to help shed those pounds? Breastfeeding. It's also important to make time for walks, with your baby in tow, whenever you can.

Gestational Diabetes

One of the most common and serious complications that can occur during pregnancy—and that occurs much more often among women who are overweight or obese—is gestational diabetes. Gestational diabetes is diabetes that is diagnosed for the first time while a woman is pregnant. It occurs in 7 to 18 percent of all pregnancies in the United States. The weight gain and hormonal changes associated with pregnancy make it hard for your body to produce the right amount of insulin to meet its needs. If you are at high risk of developing gestational diabetes because of your weight or family history, your doctor may check your blood glucose level at your first prenatal visit. Almost all other women are tested between weeks twenty-four and twenty-eight.

Untreated, gestational diabetes can lead to serious problems for your baby, including low blood sugar right after birth, breathing problems, and being born very large and with extra fat, which can make delivery dangerous for both of you. The good news is that there are steps you can take to keep it under control, including following a strict meal plan (with limits on carbohydrates and sweets), getting enough physical activity, and, in some cases, insulin injections.

Even better, the condition is usually temporary, and your blood sugar reverts to normal within six to twelve weeks of giving birth. In 5 to 10 percent of cases, though, it doesn't go away. In many of those cases, it may be that the mother already had type 2 diabetes before conception but hadn't been diagnosed yet. However, even if your diabetes disappears after you give birth, you are at risk of developing type 2 diabetes later in life. In fact, women with a history of gestational diabetes have a 35 to 60 percent chance of developing type 2 diabetes within ten years after giving birth. And it's not just about you. Your baby is also at an increased risk of becoming obese or developing diabetes.

But as we described earlier, if you developed gestational diabetes during your pregnancy, there are things you can do afterwards to reduce those odds: Lose 7 to 10 percent of your body weight; get thirty minutes of physical activity most days; and eat more whole grains, fruits, and vegetables while cutting down on calories, focusing on nutrient-dense foods, and cutting back on sugary drinks. For more on how to prevent diabetes, see chapter 3.

SUCCESS STORIES

Fortunately, there are also things you can do to reduce the odds that your child will become obese or develop type 2 diabetes, as Kerri, a forty-year-old hospital technician from Boston, would tell you.

Kerri was shocked when she developed gestational diabetes while pregnant with her son, Jake, because she didn't realize that she was at risk. She had no family history of the disease, and she didn't think of herself as overweight. "When the doctor calculated it, though, she told me I was actually on the borderline of being obese," Kerri says. "I felt good, went to classes at the gym a few times a week, didn't eat terribly. I thought I looked good, and I thought I was healthy. But I wasn't."

When Kerri underwent the routine glucose test around twenty-five weeks of pregnancy, her blood sugar was so high that her doctor immediately referred her to a specialized gestational diabetes clinic at Brigham and Women's Hospital, run by Dr. Emma Eggleston. Dr. Eggleston and her staff helped Kerri take control of her diabetes. She transformed her eating habits and began eating salad for lunch and a lean protein and vegetables for dinner each night, and made time in her busy day to walk thirty minutes before work. Although she still needed insulin to keep her glucose under control, Kerri successfully managed her gestational diabetes, and gave birth to a healthy boy who weighed seven pounds ten ounces.

Even though Kerri's blood sugar returned to normal after Jake was born, she knows that both she and Jake are at risk of developing diabetes. Because of that, Kerri and her husband, Josh, are keeping a close eye on Jake. She breast-fed him as long as she could and didn't introduce solid foods until he was six months old. Jake just turned one, and he celebrated with fruit, not birthday cake. His favorite foods are chicken, peas, and cantaloupe. As he grows, Kerri and Josh hope to continue instilling good eating habits in him and encouraging him to get a lot of exercise. Right now, though, he burns off most of his calories crawling.

Kerri is trying to get her weight under control, too. She and Josh would love to have a sibling for Jake, but they worry that Kerri would again develop gestational diabetes. She also is concerned about her own long-term health and her elevated risk of developing type 2 diabetes in just the next few years. "I don't want to be an overweight mom or a sick mom. I want to be a healthy, active mom who's here for my son for a very long time."

To Your Child's Health

Believe it or not, pregnancy is a time to influence your child's future health. Once our children enter the world, there are so many forces that are often beyond a parent's control: the foods others expose them to, the ads they see, the education they receive, and, as they get older, their own priorities and choices. (Try telling a teenager what to eat!) But the womb is a controlled environment, and the future person not yet fully formed.

Studies have shown that a mother's weight and dietary intake not only affect the development of the child in utero but can also increase the child's chances of developing obesity and diabetes down the road.

Working to get down to a healthy weight before becoming pregnant, gaining within the recommended range, eating right, getting enough activity, being tested for gestational diabetes and keeping it under control if you have it: All of these will help set your child on a course toward health. This is a wonderful opportunity to influence your child's future health, so why not seize the moment?

The Question of Surgery

You may be wondering how we've made it this far without even mentioning weight-loss surgery. Well, here's a quick rundown of the most important things you need to know about weight-loss surgery, also called bariatric surgery.

Who Is It For?

The first thing to know is that weight-loss surgery is usually advised only for people with a BMI of 40 or higher, or for those with a BMI of 35 or higher and another serious health problem, like diabetes, heart disease, or sleep apnea. You know by now that losing weight and keeping it off is incredibly difficult, and the more weight you have to lose the harder that effort is. For anyone who remains severely obese after trying multiple other approaches to weight loss, bariatric surgery may be the next step. It is a step that more than 200,000 people in this country now take each year.

Dr. David Flum, a bariatric surgeon at the University of Washington Medical Center, says:

> Some people make judgments about people who have obesity surgery. They think that they may be weak or don't have strong character, that they cop out, that they need to do an operation instead of doing the hard work of diet and exercise. But as a surgeon who deals with folks who are struggling with obesity, I've really tried to move beyond the blame game. And when you see the people who've gone through the struggle, you realize it's exactly the opposite. These are folks who have to have phenomenal determination to diet and exercise and who put their life on the line to have an operation that they can't reverse. The character it takes to effect dramatic change like that is a rare thing and something we need to celebrate.

Types of Surgery

Bariatric surgery promotes weight loss by restricting food intake. All bariatric surgery patients must make a lifelong commitment to changing the way they eat and getting regular physical activity if they want to succeed at keeping the weight off in the years after the surgery. But there are a number of different types of surgery, which all operate in different ways.

Most bariatric surgery today is performed laparoscopically—surgeons make a few small cuts through which they insert high-tech instruments and a small camera that sends a feed to a monitor and allows them to watch what they're doing. This approach creates less tissue damage, leads to fewer complications, and decreases time spent in the hospital. However, patients who weigh more than 350 pounds or have severe heart disease or other complex medical problems may need to have the surgery performed in the traditional "open" manner.

There are three types of operations most commonly offered in the

United States: adjustable gastric band, gastric bypass, and vertical sleeve gastrectomy. The adjustable gastric band is a small band that's placed around the top of the stomach to restrict the size of the opening. A balloon inside the band controls the size of the opening, and it can be inflated or deflated with saline solution to meet the changing needs of the patient over time. This procedure works primarily by decreasing food intake.

The gastric bypass, more formally known as Roux-en-Y gastric bypass, both restricts food intake and decreases absorption of food. Surgeons cut away most of the stomach, leaving just a small pouch, which they then attach to a downstream part of the small intestine. The stomach and much of the small intestine no longer come into contact with the food, which affects the release of digestive juices and certain hormones.

Finally, there's the vertical sleeve gastrectomy, which, like the gastric bypass, both restricts food intake and decreases absorption. In this procedure, most of the stomach is removed, which may decrease ghrelin (the hunger hormone), thereby decreasing appetite, as well.

Side Effects May Include . . .

No surgery is without its risks, especially when it's being performed on a high-risk population. According to Dr. Flum, "This surgery would be easy if we performed it on healthy patients." But obviously that's not the case. Dr. Flum is one of the principal investigators of the NIH's Longitudinal Assessment of Bariatric Surgery (LABS), which is looking to quantify the benefits and risks of all types of bariatric procedures. LABS researchers found that, within thirty days of surgery, 4.1 percent of patients had at least one major adverse outcome, including development of blood clots, repeat surgeries, failure to be discharged from the hospital within the month, or death. Mortality rates were low: 2.1 percent among study participants who underwent open gastric bypass, and who tended to be heavier and sicker than others in the study; 0.2 percent among those who had a laparoscopic gastric bypass; and no deaths among patients who received an adjustable gastric band. The overall death rate across all types of bariatric surgery is 0.3 percent, or 3 in 1,000.

The complications also increase as the weight of the patient increases, and with the existence of other factors such as sleep apnea or a history of blood clots. The heavier a person is, the more likely it is that there will be complications.

And then there are the long-term challenges. Since food is poorly absorbed as a result of many of these operations, people who have had bariatric surgery must always take vitamin and mineral supplements. Without supplements, they can develop nutrient deficiencies.

SUCCESS STORIES

Darrell, a sixty-three-year-old judge in Seattle, suffered quite a few complications after undergoing a laparoscopic gastric bypass a year and a half ago. But he'd do it all over again, he says, in a heartbeat. Darrell had struggled with his weight for his entire life. "I didn't make it through law school or my career as a judge by not working hard or being passionate or committed to something. But this was the one problem I could never solve. So when I finally decided to have the surgery, I looked at it as a tool to help me achieve my goals: living a life free of debilitating pain and disease, enjoying the activities I used to love, and sticking around to see my grandkids grow up."

His surgery seemed to go well, but his condition quickly deteriorated. He suffered everything from infections to kidney stones, and required multiple additional operations of various severity in order to set things right again. Today, though, he has lost almost

150 pounds, and if you were to look up "new lease on life" in the dictionary, there'd be a picture of Darrell.

He is off all three of the medications he used to take for high blood pressure, and he's off all his diabetes drugs as well, with the exception of a small dose of insulin. If he hadn't been diabetic for so long, he says, he'd probably be off insulin entirely. Even better, Darrell's playing golf with his son for the first time in a decade, spending hours bent over in his garden without all the pain, and enjoying watching his first grandson learn and grow, as his own weight decreases.

Benefits

The benefits of weight-loss surgery can be enormous. Studies have shown that the surgery results in an incredible decrease in mortality— anywhere from 23.7 to 40 percent less—when compared to similarly obese people with health problems who did not have bariatric surgery. Even ten to fifteen years after surgery, patients have reduced the development of diabetes and cardiovascular disease, and greatly improved those conditions when they already existed. As Dr. Flum puts it, when it comes to diabetes, gastric bypass in particular does something almost magical. You might think that patients' diabetes improves over the months and years after surgery, as they shed their excess weight. Amazingly, however, gastric bypass surgery can completely reverse diabetes in mere days, suggesting that there is some sort of independent mechanism contributing to the process. Obesity may cause diabetes on the way up, but weight-loss surgery improves diabetes before the patient has even lost a pound.

A BENEFIT FOR ALL OF US

The speed with which gastric bypass surgery can reverse diabetes is truly astounding, and even the world's experts can only throw out some guesses as to why it happens. But Dr. Flum, who is a researcher as well as a surgeon, is among those scientists dedicated to understanding it. "There is a set of secrets in our body that we need to understand. Secrets about why diabetes comes on and how weight loss can make it go away. We are finely tuned machines and yet, as doctors, we know so little about that tuning," he admits.

These operations are a window into understanding what that machinery is all about. And so I view every patient who has one of these operations as a way to learn about the mechanisms that are making diabetes go away. What are the mechanisms that are making hunger signals change? Because if we can bottle those things, we may have a less invasive way, a less risky way, to achieve some of these benefits without surgery, allowing us all to live healthier and happier lives.

Finding the Right Surgeon

The final thing to keep in mind if you're considering bariatric surgery for yourself or for a loved one is that all surgeons, and all hospitals, are not created equal. Practice makes perfect, so when talking to any prospective surgeon, be sure to ask how many times he or she has performed the procedure. If the answer is a two-digit number, you may want to continue your search.

It's also important to ask what kind of support groups the program offers. Talking to people who have undergone the same procedure is the best way of arriving at a full understanding of the risks, side effects, and rewards of bariatric surgery before you sign up for it. And a group of like-minded folks who know what you're going through can help you make it through the often challenging time people have after surgery as they learn to adjust to their new bodies.

As for the hospitals, the American Society for Metabolic & Bariatric Surgery awards the ones with the best surgical outcomes the designation "Center of Excellence." These programs are the most reputable; the most highly regarded by others in the field; and the most likely to provide you with the additional support you need, both leading up to and following surgery, in order for you to succeed. You can search for a surgeon at a Center of Excellence nearby at http://asmbs.org/member-search.

Footing the Bill

Bariatric surgery isn't cheap. The procedures, on average, cost between twenty thousand and twenty-five thousand dollars. Private medical insurance often covers the surgery, especially if you have concurrent conditions like diabetes or heart disease. Medicare may also cover it if you have at least one obesity-linked health problem and if approved surgeons and facilities deem the procedure suitable for your medical condition. Contact your insurance provider to find out more.

Additional Reading

Bringing It to the Table by Wendell Berry (2009)

Catching Fire: How Cooking Made Us Human by Richard Wrangham (2009)

The End of Food by Paul Roberts (2009)

The End of Overeating by David A. Kessler, M.D. (2009)

The Evolution of Obesity by Michael L. Power and Jay Schulkin (2009)

Fat, Fate, and Disease: Why We Are Losing the War Against Obesity and Chronic Disease by Peter Gluckman and Mark Hanson (2012)

Fat Land by Greg Critser (2003)

The Fattening of America by Eric A. Finkelstein and Laurie Zuckerman (2008)

Food Politics by Marion Nestle (2002, revised 2007)

Food Rules: An Eater's Manual by Michael Pollan (2009)

Free for All: Fixing School Food in America by Janet Poppendieck (2011)

The Hundred Year Diet: America's Voracious Appetite for Losing Weight by Susan Yager (2010)

In Defense of Food: An Eater's Manifesto by Michael Pollan (2009)

Additional Reading

Mindless Eating: Why We Eat More Than We Think by Brian Wansink (2010)

Mismatch: Why Our World No Longer Fits Our Bodies by Peter Gluckman and Mark Hanson (2006)

Prescription for a Healthy Nation: A New Approach to Improving Our Lives by Fixing Our Everyday World by Tom Farley and Deborah Cohen (2006)

Rethinking Thin: The New Science of Weight Loss—and the Myths and Realities of *Dieting* by Gina Kolata (2008)

What to Eat by Marion Nestle (2006)

The World Is Fat: The Fads, Trends, Policies, and Products that Are Fattening the Human Race by Barry Popkin (2009)

[To see attribution for the quotations marked with an asterisk, please go to hbo.com/theweightofthenation.]